total BODY PLAN

KU-441-112

By Lucy Wyndham-Read

Photography **Tom Miles,** Food and Drink Photography **Danny Bird**

Hair & Make-up **Ryutaro @ Eta Management using L'Oréal Tecni-Art**

Cover model **Hollie Simmons @ WAthletic**

Art Editor **Jo Gurney**

Illustrations **Martina Farrow, New Division Illustrations**

Subeditor **John Murphy**

Editor **Mary Comber**

Advertising **Katie Wood katie_wood@dennis.co.uk**

Advertising **Matt Wakefield matt_wakefield@dennis.co.uk**

Editorial Director **Pete Muir**

Digital Production Manager **Nicky Baker**

Bookazine Manager **Dharmesh Mistry**

Operations Director **Robin Ryan**

Managing Director of Advertising **Julian Lloyd-Evans**

Newstrade Director **David Barker**

Chief Operating Officer **Brett Reynolds**

Group Finance Director **Ian Leggett**

Chief Executive **James Tye**

Chairman **Felix Dennis**

With thanks to **Amazon** amazon.co.uk

Casall www.casall.com, **Wellicious** www.wellicious.com

Asics Trainer www.asics.co.uk

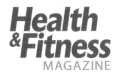 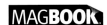

Total Body Plan ISBN 1-907779-95-7

To license this product please contact Hannah Heagney on +44 (0) 20 7907 6134 or email hannah_heagney@dennis.co.uk

While every care was taken during the production of this Magbook, the publishers cannot be held responsible for the accuracy of the information or any consequence arising from it. Dennis Publishing takes no responsibility for the companies advertising in this Magbook.

The paper used within this Magbook is produced from sustainable fibre, manufactured by mills with a valid chain of custody.

Printed at BGP

The health and fitness information presented in this book is an educational resource and is not intended as a substitute for medical advice. Consult your doctor or healthcare professional before performing any of the exercises described in this book or any other exercise programme, particularly if you are pregnant, or if you are elderly or have chronic or recurring medical conditions. Do not attempt any of the exercises while under the influence of alcohol or drugs. Discontinue any exercise that causes you pain or severe discomfort and consult a medical expert. Neither the author of the information nor the producer nor distributors of such information make any warranty of any kind in regard to the content of the information presented in this book.

To subscribe to Health & Fitness magazine call **0844 844 0081** or go to **www.healthandfitnessonline.co.uk**

CHANGE

YOUR REFLECTION

Diet Protein is arguably the most sophisticated diet protein shake available today. Reflex Nutrition have used the latest advances in protein and weight loss technology to bring you a product that's specifically designed to help you achieve a healthy, well defined and toned body.

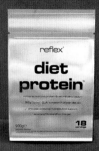

RRP £32.99
900g - 18 x 50g servings

> One serving of Reflex Diet Protein provides 3.2 grams of Clarinol™ CLA, a research based dose proven to help reduce body fat primarily in the abdomen and particularly in women, the legs.

> Each serving of Reflex Diet Protein is packed with additional diet support. Green Tea extract is added for its long standing reputation for aiding dieters.

> Diet Protein contains no added sugar or maltodextrin. It's perfect for dieters wanting to restrict their carbohydrate content.

> Diet Protein comes in a variety of mouthwatering flavours. All of which have been up against a taste test panel to ensure that they are the best tasting diet shakes on the market.

Find out more about our products at:

www.reflex-nutrition.com

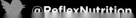

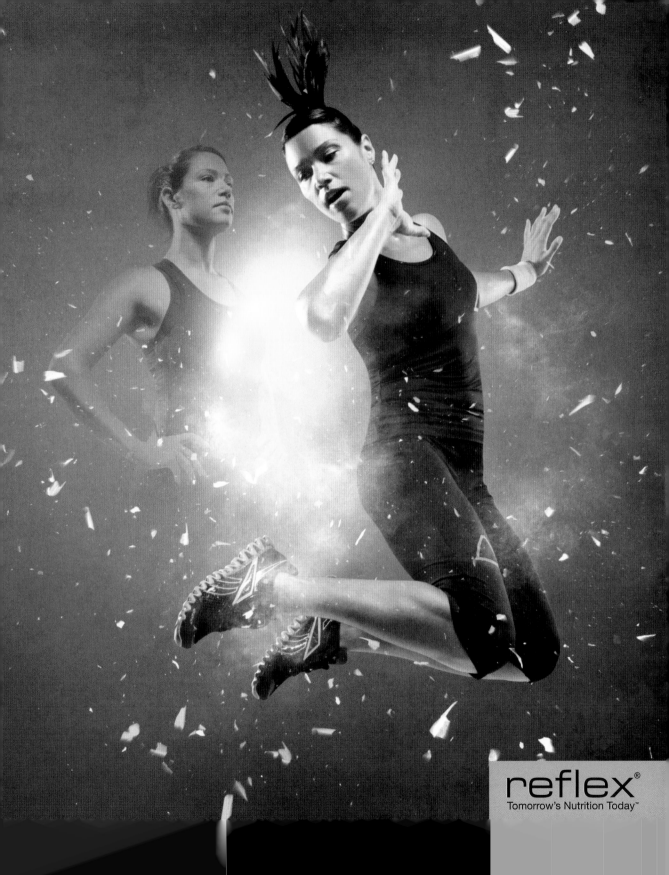

reflex®
Tomorrow's Nutrition Today™

Contents...

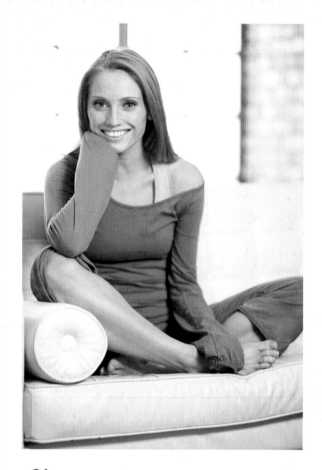

About the author

Lucy Wyndham-Read has more than 17 years' experience of health, fitness and nutrition. She has written several books on women's fitness, as well as being a regular on TV and radio, giving advice on how women can stay fit.

She began her career in the Army and is now a qualified personal trainer, specialising in antenatal and postnatal fitness, weight loss, nutrition, children's health and exercise. She is also founder of lwrfitness.com. Lucy's passion is showing women that exercise can be easy. She has helped hundreds of women to lose weight and get in shape. Her motivation is infectious and she believes that we can all find some form of exercise we enjoy.

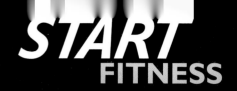

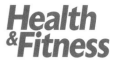
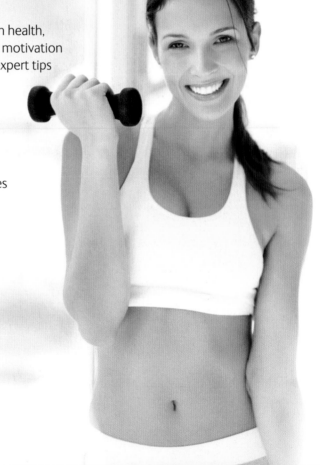
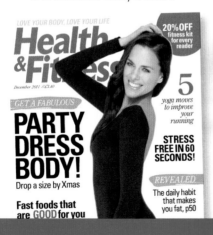

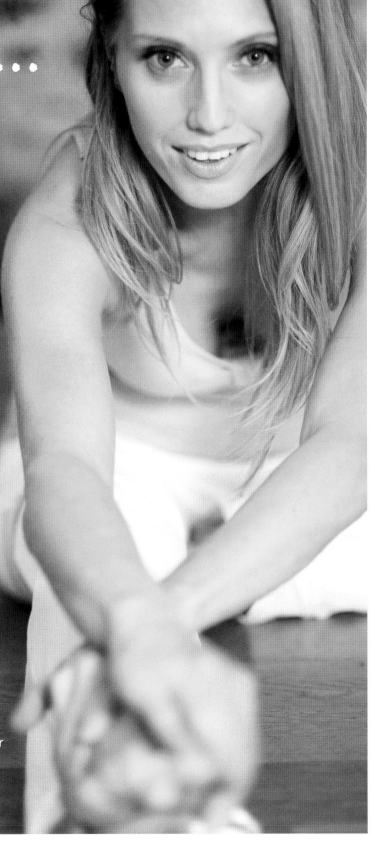

Lucy says...

Over my 17 years as a personal trainer, I have heard the same thing from clients time and again: 'I can never find the time to exercise.' This is why I have spent years creating effective workouts for women that can be done at home in no time and that are guaranteed to get the results you want.

Women are busier than ever juggling family, home and work. It can be hard to squeeze in a session at the gym or a Tums 'n' Bums class. The good news is that you can do an effective workout in less than 15 minutes. You can train at home and increase your energy levels, lose fat and tone up those areas that are most important to women: legs, tummy, bum, arms and bust.

It's exciting to show women how simple it can be to start getting fit. As soon as you start feeling fitter you won't want to stop. I believe that we can all find 15 minutes, and that it will be time well spent, because fitness is not only great for your health, it is also the best anti-ageing weapon there is.

A good exercise and diet programme should be simple, fun and quick. After six weeks of this plan, you will be looking younger, your body will be slimmer and firmer and you'll be glowing with vitality.

What you'll get
the benefits

Once upon a time, everyone led active lives and ate only natural foods. But that was before the inventions of cars, escalators, TVs, computers, microwaves, ready meals, hydrogenated fats and the supersize meal deal.

Modern lifestyles make it easy to avoid exercise and healthy eating, so you need a good reason spend valuable time exercising and cooking meals from scratch. And here is where I persuade you that doing this six-week plan will reap significant benefits.

Exercise is not simply about weight loss. Even naturally slim people need to exercise regularly to maintain a strong heart, help keep joints flexible, reduced stress and prevent medical conditions such as diabetes and cancer.

It doesn't matter how old you are – we all need to exercise to keep our bones, joints and muscles strong, which includes the most important muscle of all: the heart. Regular exercise will help to keep your blood pressure down, reduce cholesterol, maintain a healthy body weight and is especially important for women to help prevent osteoporosis.

Every time you exercise or eat a healthy meal you will feel the benefits straightaway. Your body floods with feel-good hormones that make you energised and optimistic, and this creates a positive spiral, because the better you feel, the more confident you feel, the more you want to continue exercising. It doesn't take long before you start to look healthy and radiant.

20 benefits of this plan...

* You will have more energy
* You will have more confidence
* You will lose weight
* You will tone up
* You will look glowing
* You will simply feel better
* You will sleep better
* You will drop a dress size
* Your will tone up your legs
* You will define your waist
* You will lift your bust
* You will increase the amount of calories you burn
* You will tone your legs
* You will look younger
* You will sculpt your arms
* You will reduce cellulite
* You will slow down the ageing process
* You will improve your health
* You will be more resilient to illness
* You will be able to make exercise a lifetime habit

Your body
the target areas

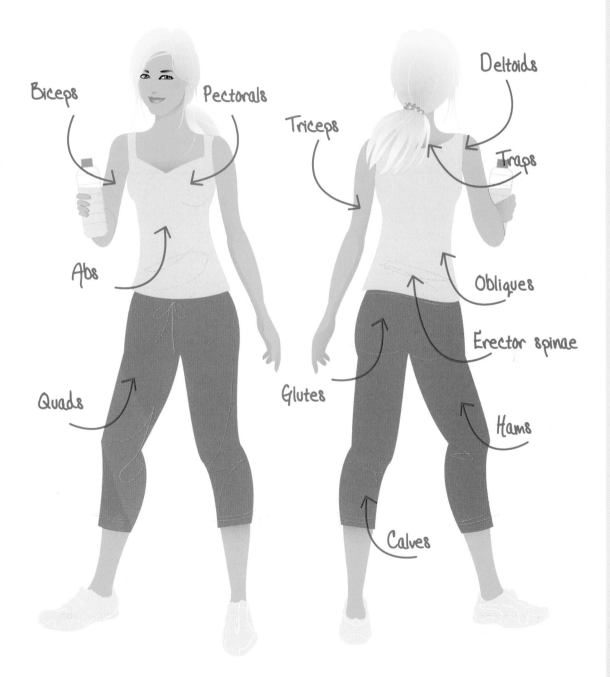

Biceps

Pectorals

Triceps

Deltoids

Traps

Abs

Obliques

Erector spinae

Quads

Glutes

Hams

Calves

What you'll

the kit list

You can get started on this programme straightaway, without having to buy expensive home gym kit or pay for a gym membership. If you want to invest in a few useful items, such as hand weights or an exercise mat, then that's great, but you can easily make do with stuff that you can find around the house.

Mat or towel For the floor exercises, a thick towel will be good enough to protect your joints and back when performing moves.

Hand weights or water bottles Some of the circuit exercises require these to provide resistance for your muscles. Hand weights are the neatest option, but you can use plastic milk bottles as these tend to have handles so they're great for getting a good grip. As you get fitter you can increase the weight by filling them with more water.

Chair Any chair will do. It will come into play during some of the circuits.

Cushion or pillow This will mainly be used for squeezing between your palms or thighs to create muscle tension.

Clock with a second hand All the exercises are done on a timed basis so it's useful to have a big clock face with a second hand so you can easily see when your 60 seconds is up and it's time to move on to the next exercise.

Trainers You will need these for the aerobic workouts. They should have good cushioning, so it's worth investing in a decent pair if you don't already own something suitable.

Sports bra This is a recommendation rather than a necessity. But a good sports bra is worth the money because it can prevent sagging breasts as a result of over-stretched ligaments. Make sure you buy one that fits properly.

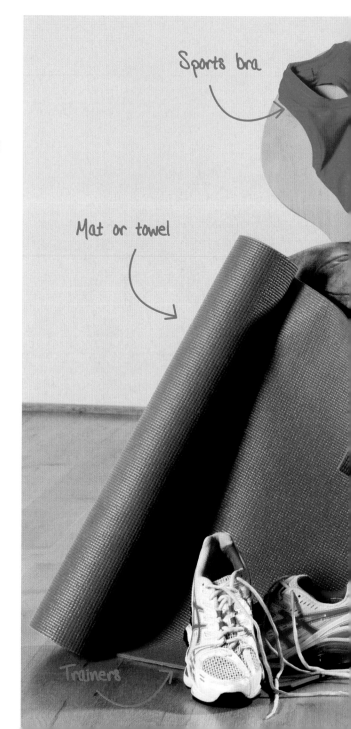

Sports bra

Mat or towel

Trainers

need

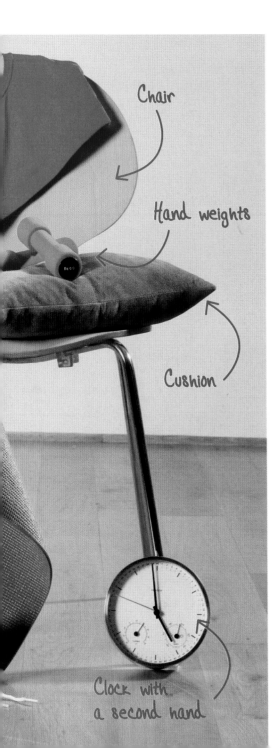

Chair

Hand weights

Cushion

Clock with
a second hand

Things to remember...

Before you do your exercises make sure
you stick to the following rules

 Do...

... drink plenty of water

... put on some motivating music and get into
a positive frame of mind

... always warm up

... follow the form guides in the book closely

... start gently and build up slowly

... stay safe by wearing bright and reflective
clothing when exercising outdoors

... always let someone know where you are going

... avoid taking alleyways or always doing the
same route at the same time on the same day

... always take a phone with you when outside

... finish off exercising with your stretches

Don't...

... train on an empty stomach

... exercise if you are not feeling well

... keep exercising if you feel pain of any kind

... worry if you have the occasional day where you
can't complete your routine. Stay focused and just
start again the next day

Test yourself
see how fit you are

One of the best ways to stay motivated is to see for yourself the changes that your fitness programme is achieving. When you can see that you have less body fat, that your limbs feel stronger and firmer and that you have more energy and endurance, it makes you want to continue with the programme and see even more good results. Before you start your six-week plan take these simple fitness tests. Then take them again after three weeks of following the programme so you can see how you've improved. They will give you a clear indication of what you can achieve if you stick with the plan through to the end of week six.

1 Warm-up

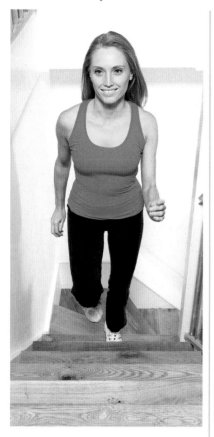

Start by marching on the spot for two minutes, or jog up and down the stairs, to get your muscles warmed up. After you have completed the three tests described to the right, finish off by completing your full set of stretches as shown on page 19.

2 Lower body test

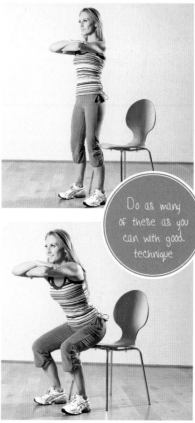

Do as many of these as you can with good technique

Stand in front of a chair with your feet hip-width apart, cross your arms over your chest and, keeping your body weight over your heels, bend your knees until the backs of your thighs touch the chair seat. Take four seconds to lower and two seconds to stand.

3 Upper body test

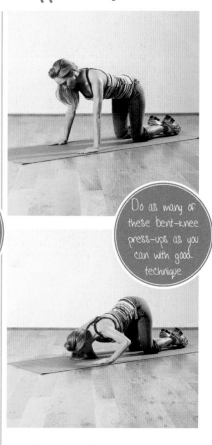

Do as many of these bent-knee press-ups as you can with good technique

Kneel with your hands just ahead of your shoulders, arms straight. Your body should form a straight line from your head to your hips. Bend your elbows to lower your body until your chest is about three inches from the floor, then push back up to the start.

> Write down the results from each of these tests so you can compare them in three weeks time

4 Abdominal test

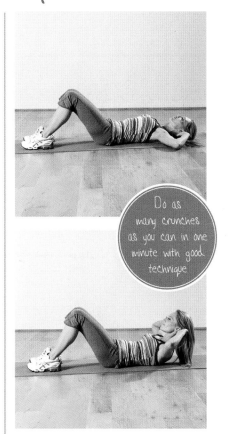

> Do as many crunches as you can in one minute with good technique

Lie on your back with knees bent and feet flat on the floor. Place your hands behind your head, fingers touching but not clasped. Use your abdominal muscles to lift your shoulders off the floor and curl your chest towards your knees. Lower yourself slowly back to the floor.

Measure up
CHECK YOUR SIZES

When it comes to measuring how well you are progressing throughout the six-week programme, I'm a big fan of the tape measure rather than the weighing scales. The tape measure will reflect the changes in your body shape, which is the main aim of this programme. After six weeks you should have a narrower waist , a lifted bottom, a toned bust and slimmer thighs.

I recommend that you measure at the beginning of the programme then at the halfway point. This will keep you motivated to do even better by the six-week stage.

If you still like to jump on the scales, my advice is to use them sparingly. A constant weight can be demotivating, even if your body shape is changing all the time. Always weigh or measure yourself on the same day at the same time, for example a Monday morning before breakfast.

Bust
Measure over your nipple line.

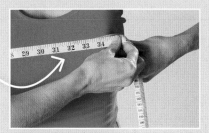

Waist
You're at your narrowest around your belly button.

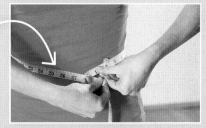

Bottom
Loop the tape round at your widest point.

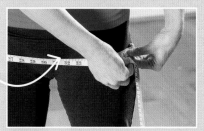

Thigh
Measure your right thigh a quarter of a way down your upper leg.

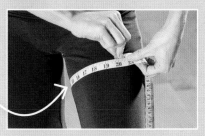

How it works
the six-week plan explained

The programme is very simple to follow. Each week you will do three aerobic sessions and three circuits, with a rest day on Sunday. Each of the sessions takes no more than 15 minutes, so they are easy to fit into a busy day and you don't need expensive gyms or acres of space to do them.

Aerobic plans

These involve walking, running, jumping – anything that gets your heart rate up. This is important for keeping your heart and lungs healthy, and it's also a great way to burn off body fat.

As with any form of exercise, it is important that you work out to the correct intensity. For example, a 15-minute slow walk won't do you any harm but you won't get the desired results of weight loss and increased fitness, so you need to be pushing yourself harder. On the other hand, pushing too hard will only end up with you hitting exhaustion and being unable to complete your session.

There is an easy way of gauging the correct level to exercise at, and this is known as The Perceived Rate of Exertion (see opposite), which we will use throughout this programme.

Every week I have designed you a new plan. This keeps the programme full of variety so you never get bored.

Circuits

Circuits are resistance exercises performed one after the other with no rest in between. This method will keep your heart rate high and save you time. Each circuit in the six-week plan consists of five exercises, and they will focus on those areas that women want to keep honed and toned: bust, abs, arms, bottom and thighs. As well as toning your muscles, circuits help to burn off fat even after you've finished, because they raise your metabolism. Circuits will also help to keep your bones strong, which for women is vital to prevent osteoporosis.

Each circuit routine will take just five minutes, plus your warm-up and stretching time. If you have more time – and more energy – then you can repeat each circuit twice.

Meal plans

Diet is obviously vital to help you lose fat while providing enough energy to perform the exercises and enough vitamins and minerals to stay healthy. The plan I've created is easy to follow and quick to prepare. At the end of each section is a shopping list so you can stock up for each week. You don't have to calorie-count or weigh all your food – that can get complicated. Aim to stick to the portion sizes on page 34 so that you are not tempted to overeat.

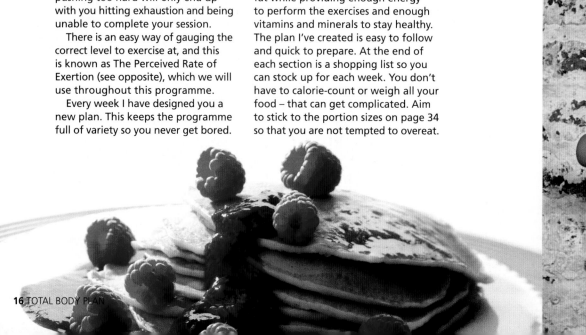

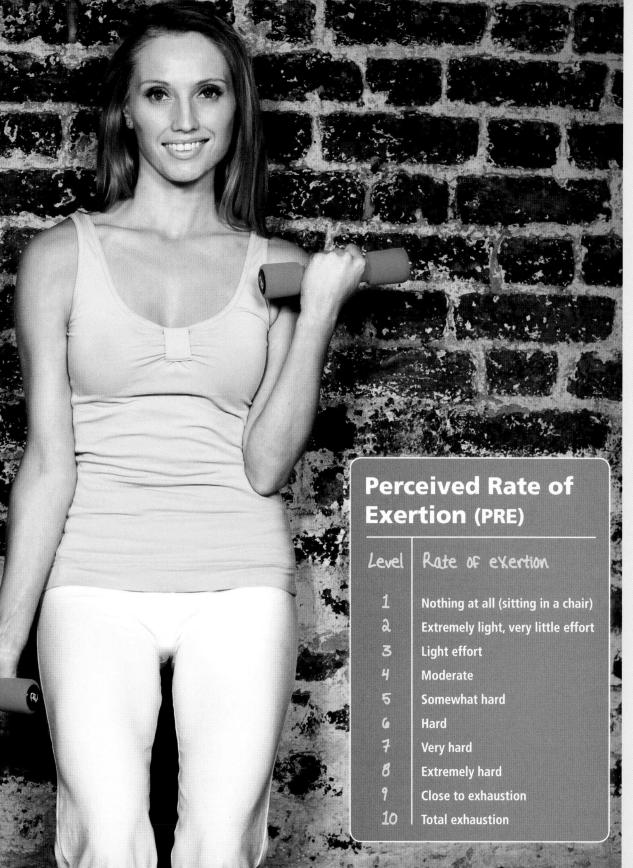

Perceived Rate of Exertion (PRE)

Level	Rate of exertion
1	Nothing at all (sitting in a chair)
2	Extremely light, very little effort
3	Light effort
4	Moderate
5	Somewhat hard
6	Hard
7	Very hard
8	Extremely hard
9	Close to exhaustion
10	Total exhaustion

Warm-up
and stretching

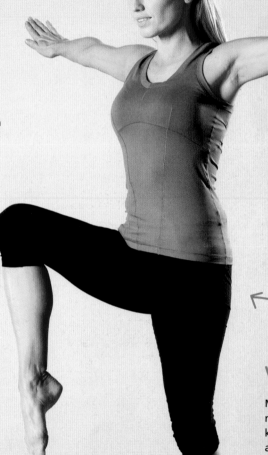

I t is always important to warm up before you do any form of exercise. A warm-up helps prevent injuries due to cold muscles and it will improve the range of movement throughout your body, making exercise more effective. It also prepares you mentally for the exercises to come.

Stretching after your sessions will help to lengthen tight muscles and flush out toxins, making you more flexible and helping your recovery.

For all the aerobic plans, the warm-up is included within the set routine and you will only need to do the stretches at the end of the workout. For your circuit training, I recommend that you always spend between two and three minutes warming up, starting gently and building up your range of movement.

Warm-up

March up and down the room for a few minutes, keeping your knees high and circling your arms out at the sides.

Hamstring stretch

Rest both your hands on your supporting leg and feel the stretch all the way through the back of the straight leg. Hold for ten seconds on each leg.

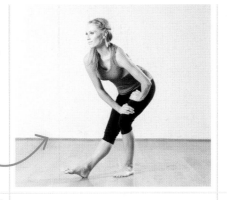

Quads stretch

Stand with good posture, raise one leg behind you and hold the foot while pushing your hips forward. Keep the supporting knee slightly bent. Hold for ten seconds on each leg.

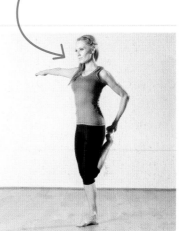

Chest stretch

Stand with good posture and hold your hands behind your back. Lift your shoulders up and press your arms back to feel the stretch in your chest. Hold for ten seconds.

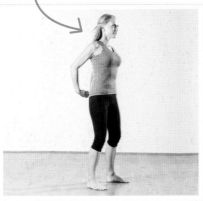

Calf stretch

Step back with one leg. Keep the leg straight and the heel down, with both feet pointing forwards. Rest your hands on the bent leg and feel the stretch in the back leg. Hold for ten seconds on each leg.

Back stretch

Stand with good posture. Keep your knees soft and your tummy pulled in. Hold your arms in front of you as if you are hugging a big beach ball. Feel the stretch in your back. Hold for ten seconds.

Triceps stretch

Stand up straight, knees slightly bent and tummy pulled in. Lift one arm up and bend it behind your head, aiming to get your hand between your shoulder blades. Gently pull on your elbow with your other arm. Hold for ten seconds on each arm.

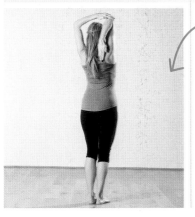

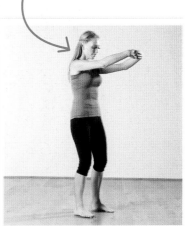

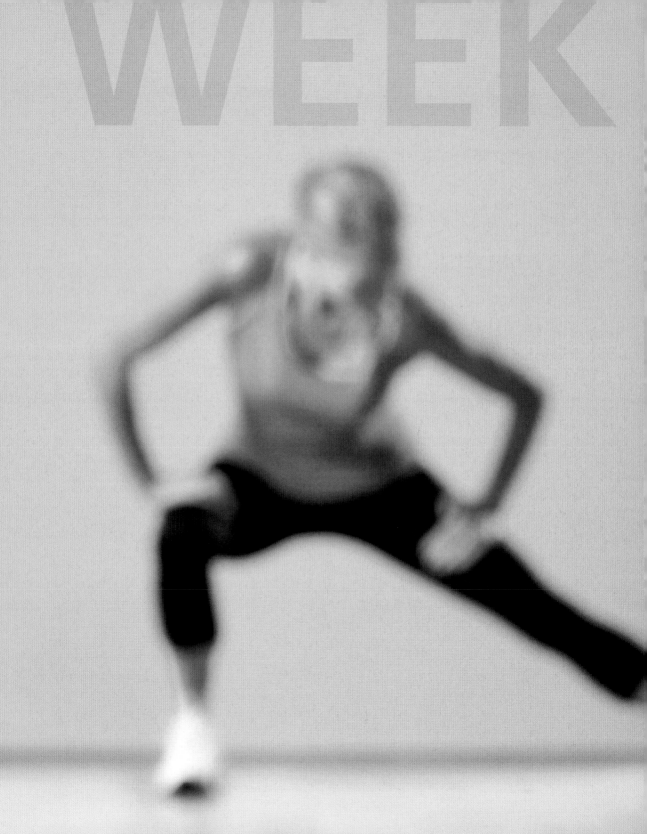

WEEK

ONE

'You are never too old to start looking younger'

WEEK ONE
the plan...

Monday Aerobic 15-minute inch-loss walk see opposite

Tuesday 1 x home circuit see p24

Wednesday Aerobic 15-minute inch-loss walk

Thursday 1 x home circuit

Friday Aerobic 15-minute inch-loss walk

Saturday 2 x home circuits

Sunday Rest

TOP TIP
To really tone up your arms, walk with hand weights or simply fill up two small bottles of water. This will not only banish bingo wings but will burn off extra calories

Aerobic
15-minute inch-loss walk

In Week One we will be walking off those extra pounds. This innovative workout can be done in just 15 minutes and will help to melt away any excess fat and tone up those troublesome areas such as the arms, bottom, tummy, hips and thighs. We will also be adding an abdominal workout to this walk so you can be toning your waist without a single sit-up.

Simply follow the chart (right) and ensure that you work to the correct level of perceived rate of exertion (see p17), as this will guarantee you results.

How to power walk
* Always walk with good posture. Keep your shoulders, hips and ankles in a vertical line, with your shoulders relaxed.
* As you walk keep your knees soft.
* Always land on your heel and push off from the front of your foot.
* Bend your elbows to about 90°. To add an abdominal workout to your walk, simply pull your belly button in tight towards your spine and hold. This will engage the deepest abdominal muscles and help to define your waist.

Time (mins)	Exercise	Perceived rate of exertion
0–2	Walk at gentle pace to help you warm up	4
2–4	Walk briskly, taking long strides and swinging your arms in an exaggerated fashion	5
4–5	Walk as fast as you can	6
5–6	Walk at moderate pace, but focus on keeping your belly button pulled in tight to your spine	5
6–8	Walk as fast as you can	6
8–9	Walk at moderate pace but focus on keeping your belly button pulled in tight to your spine	5
9–10	March on the spot lifting your knees high. Work your abs by keeping them pulled in as you march	5
10–11	Walk as fast as you can	6
11–12	Walk at moderate pace, but focus on keeping your belly button pulled in tight to your spine	5
12–13	Walk as fast as you can	6
13–15	Walk at medium pace, slowing gently towards the finish	4

Home circuits
Just ten minutes

Start by warming up for two to three minutes (see p18), then perform the following five exercises in order. Do each exercise for one minute before moving straight on to the next with no rest in between. Once you've finished, spend two minutes doing some stretching (see p19)

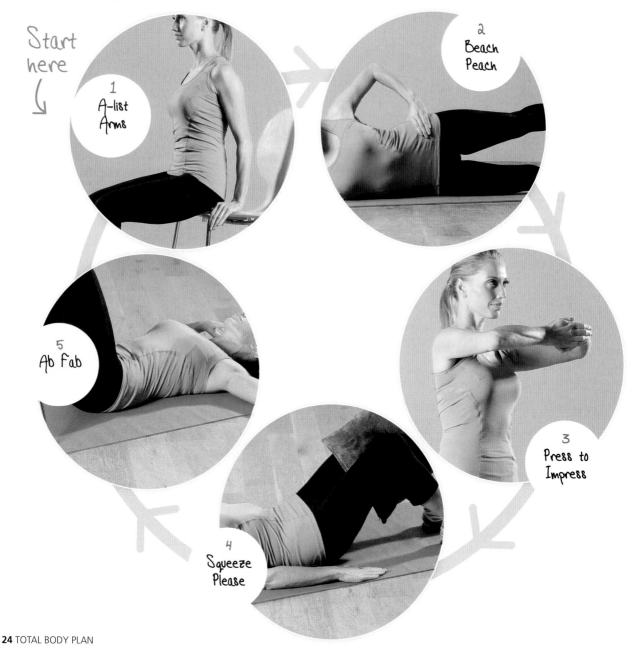

Start here

1 A-list Arms

2 Beach Peach

3 Press to Impress

4 Squeeze Please

5 Ab Fab

Exercise one

A-list Arms

What it does

This exercise targets that problematic area often referred to as the 'bingo wings'. The move tones up the backs of your upper arms, or triceps.

How to do it

Sit on the edge of a chair, hands hip-distance apart and fingertips facing your toes. Support your weight, then slip off the chair and lower yourself towards the floor by bending your elbows only. Make sure your elbows stay pointing towards the back wall as you lower down. Then slowly push back to the start, keeping your back close to the edge of the chair.

Tip: As you become fitter you can up the intensity of this exercise by placing your feet further from the chair

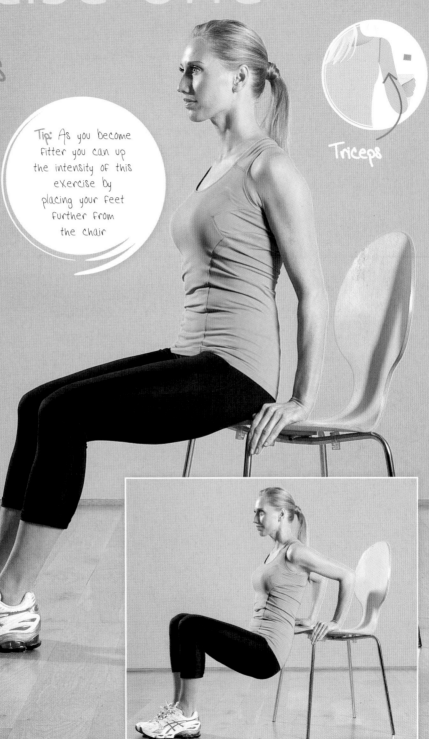

Triceps

25

Exercise two

Beach Peach

What it does

This will work deep into your abdominal muscles, while giving your bottom a lift and great overall tone.

How to do it

Lie on your mat, on your right side, so your body is in a straight line. With your lower arm supporting your head and your other hand resting on your top hip, slowly lift the top leg so your foot is higher than your hip and you have your toes pointed.

Now very slowly squeeze your bottom muscles to take your leg several inches behind you, making sure you keep the rest of your body perfectly still. Hold for a second then bring the leg back to the start.

Repeat this for 30 seconds on one leg then change sides to work the other leg.

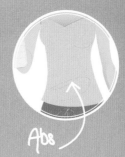

Abs

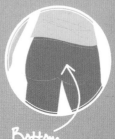

Bottom

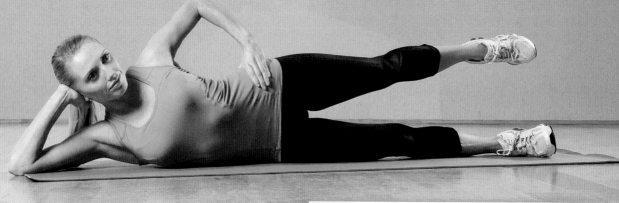

Tip: For best results keep this exercise slow and controlled with no jerky movements

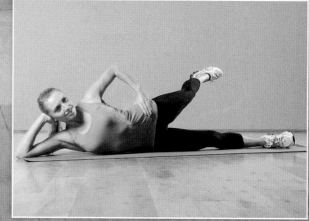

Exercise three

Press to Impress

What it does

This is such a simple exercise but it's highly effective because it helps to strengthen the muscles that support the chest, giving your bust a lift.

How to do it

Stand with good posture, knees slightly bent, abdominals pulled in tight. Press the palms of your hands together at chest height and hold for a slow count of five, release and repeat. Keep doing this for one minute, maintaining good posture throughout.

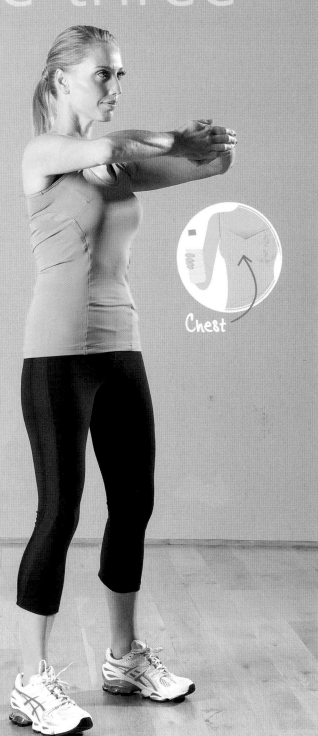

Chest

Tip: Focus on using your pectorals (chest muscles) to squeeze your hands together

Exercise four

Squeeze Please

What it does

This exercise focuses on your inner thigh muscles, helping to make your legs more shapely. The harder you squeeze, the better the results…

How to do it

Lie on your back on a towel or mat on the floor. Bend your knees and place a pillow between them. Let your upper body and arms stay relaxed on the floor. Now simply squeeze the cushion as hard as you can by pressing your knees together. Hold this squeeze for a three count then slowly release and repeat. Ensure you squeeze as hard as you can each time. Repeat this for one minute.

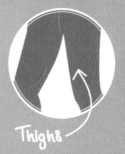

Thighs

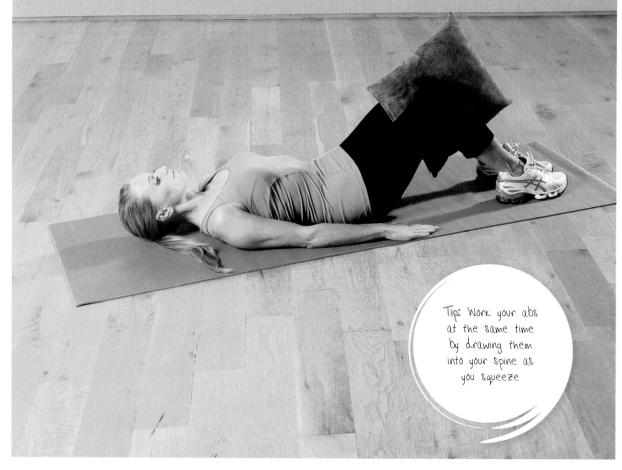

Tip: Work your abs at the same time by drawing them into your spine as you squeeze

Exercise five

Ab Fab

What it does
One of the classic abdominal exercises. Having your legs on the chair works your muscles that bit harder.

How to do it
Lie on your back on a mat or towel with your feet resting on a chair. Your legs should be bent at a 90° angle. Place your fingertips on either side of your head and look up towards the ceiling. Slowly lift your head and shoulders off the floor and hold for a few seconds, keeping your belly button pulled in tight to your spine, then slowly lower yourself to the start.

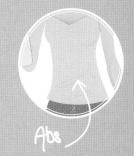

Abs

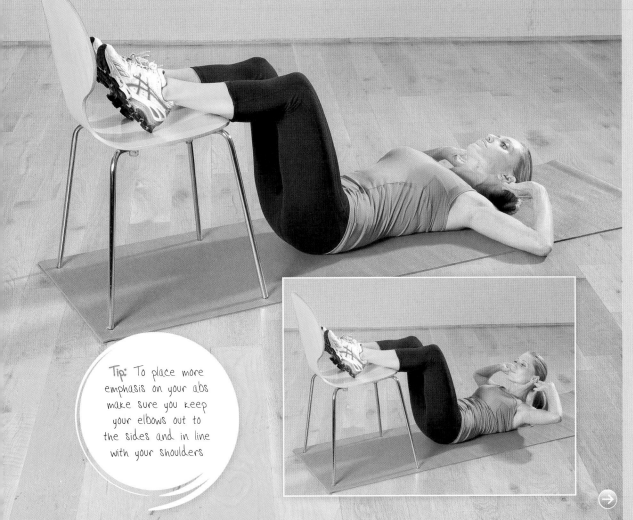

Tip: To place more emphasis on your abs make sure you keep your elbows out to the sides and in line with your shoulders

29

tuck in...

Monday	Tuesday

Breakfast
Energy-boosting smoothie
(see p35)

Mid-morning snack
150g pot of low-fat yoghurt

Lunch
Medium-sized jacket potato
with hummus and a squeeze
of lemon

Mid-afternoon snack
3 ham slices wrapped
around asparagus spears

Dinner
Baked skinless chicken
breast topped with pesto,
mixed roasted vegetables

Breakfast
2 slices of
wholemeal
toast with plum
tomatoes

Mid-morning snack
Sliced peppers with
cottage cheese

Lunch
Three-bean soup with
sprinkling of toasted seeds

Mid-afternoon snack
Banana with handful
of raisins

Dinner
Lean grilled beef steak
with green vegetables

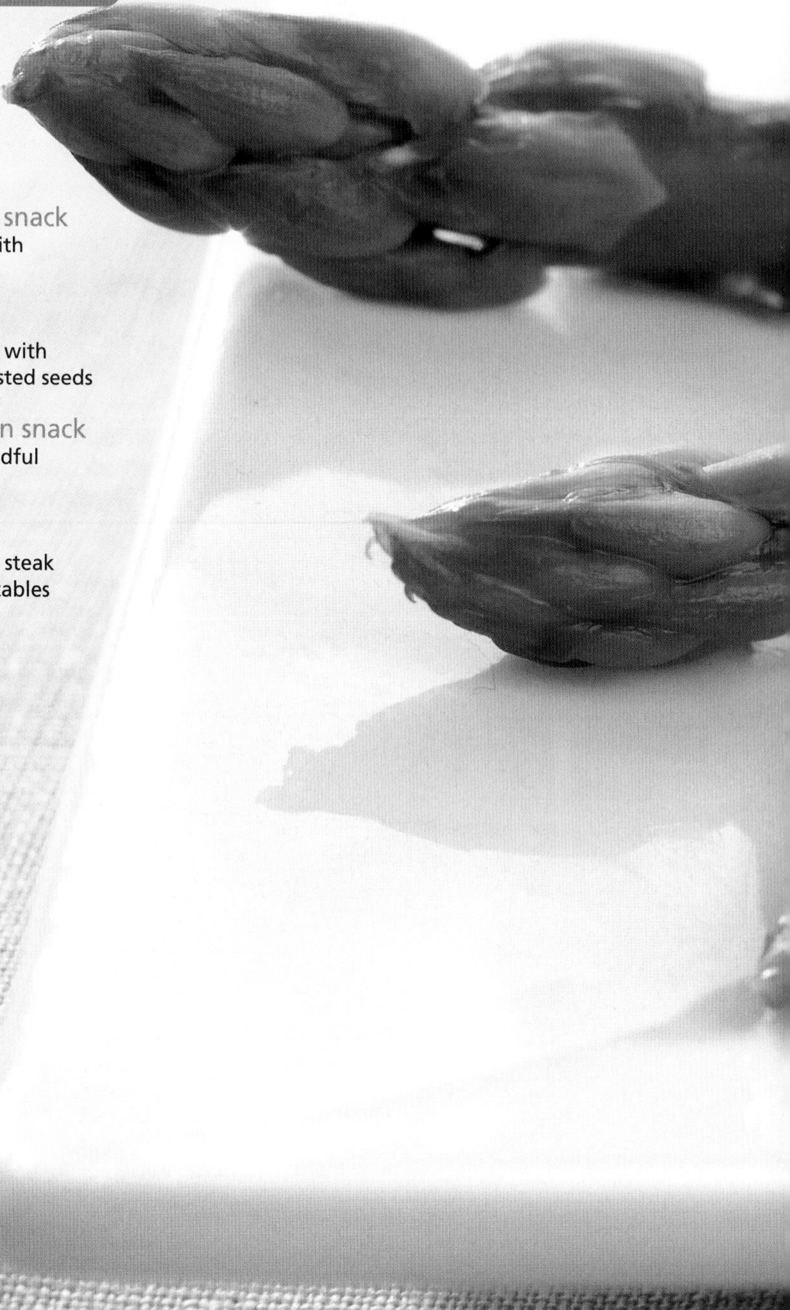

Drink lots of water

Drinking up to two litres a
day will keep you hydrated
and aid organ function so
you stay healthy and
young-looking

Wednesday

Breakfast
2 eggs scrambled on 2 pieces of wholemeal toast

Mid-morning snack
4 carrot sticks and hummus

Lunch
Small chicken salad with avocado, banana

Mid-afternoon snack
Sugar-free protein bar

Dinner
Spaghetti Bolognese – use wholemeal spaghetti and lean mince

Thursday

Breakfast
Porridge with a sprinkling of berries and seeds

Mid-morning snack
Large rice cake with avocado

Lunch
2 mini wholemeal pittas stuffed with salad leaves, sliced cucumber, tomatoes and avocado, topped with tuna

Mid-afternoon snack
Hard-boiled egg with raw carrots

Dinner
Grilled white fish with a drizzle of lemon, olive oil and herbs, served with green vegetables

Friday	Saturday	Sunday

Breakfast
Energy-boosting smoothie (see p35)

Mid-morning snack
2 Ryvitas with ham slices and cucumber

Lunch
Wholemeal wrap with avocado, tomato and low-fat mozzarella

Mid-afternoon snack
Handful of nuts and raisins

Dinner
Poached salmon fillet with leeks and green vegetables

Breakfast
Oatmeal pancake with mixed berries

Mid-morning snack
Large rice cake with small slice of low-fat cheese and pickle

Lunch
Sardines on toast

Mid-afternoon snack
Sliced cucumber, carrots and peppers with a hummus dip

Dinner
Stir-fry vegetables with rice noodles and 1tbsp soy sauce

Breakfast
Poached egg on toast, grapefruit

Mid-morning snack
150g pot of low-fat yoghurt

Lunch
Brown rice salad with chopped red onion, cherry tomatoes, kidney beans and chickpeas

Mid-afternoon snack
Toasted crumpet with a drizzle of honey

Dinner
Chicken breast served on couscous with ratatouille

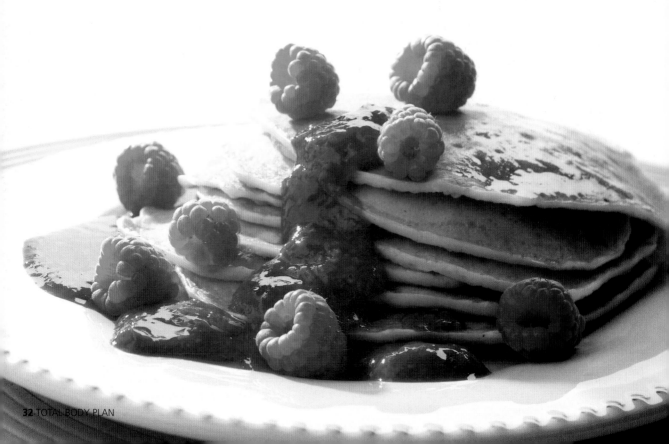

Shopping list

Wholemeal pittas, bread, wraps, spaghetti
Brown rice
Rice noodles
Couscous
Crumpets, for toasting
Low-fat milk, yoghurts, cottage cheese, mozzarella, hard cheese
Hummus
Honey
Tins of sardines, tuna, three-bean soup, tomatoes
Ryvita
Rice cakes
Oatmeal
Oats
Raisins
Nuts, mixed seeds
Fruit/veg: asparagus, avocado, bananas, carrots, cherry tomatoes
cucumber, frozen berries, grapefruit, jacket potatoes, leeks, lemon,
peppers, green vegetables, sweet potatoes
Ham slices
Lean beef steak
Salmon fillets
Chicken breasts
White fish
Lean mince
Eggs
Pickles
Pesto
Soy sauce
Sugar-free protein bar

Food facts
Size matters

I s it surprising that obesity is at epidemic proportions in the UK, when these days many food portions are triple the size they used to be? The bigger the portion the quicker the weight gain.

Clever marketing and confusing food packaging mean that it's easy to pile on the calories, even when you think you don't eat a lot. That morning coffee with the girls can seem pretty innocent until you learn that a large latte with mocha and a little whipped cream can contain as much as 360 calories – nearly a fifth or your daily allowance.

Women are recommended to take in around 2,000 calories each day to maintain a steady weight. So if you are looking to shed a few pounds, then you'll need to eat fewer than 2,000 calories a day. A simple way of doing this is swapping your dinner plate for a side plate, as this will encourage you not to eat large portions.

As a general rule, with cheese and dairy have a portion that is no bigger than the size of a matchbox. With meat and fish your portion should be the size of a pack of playing cards. And carbohydrates such as brown rice, couscous, pasta, sweet potatoes, grains and pulses should be in portions the size of the playing cards and matchbox together. As for fruit and vegetables, this is the one time you can supersize with impunity. Fill your plate!

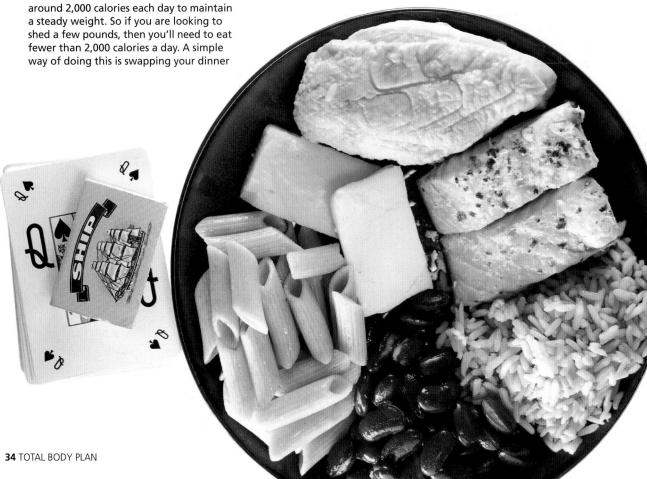

Blend it
Energy-boosting smoothie

This is a great smoothie to have for breakfast because it will keep your energy levels high throughout the day, thanks to its slow-release carbs. Plus it's quick and yummy

Ingredients
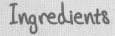

* Banana
* 150g pot of low-fat yoghurt
* 3tbsp soya milk
* 2 heaped tbsp porridge oats
* Drizzle of maple syrup

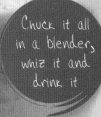

Chuck it all in a blender, whiz it and drink it

Look great
All-year holiday glow

We all know that sunbathing is not good for the skin. It can make your skin age prematurely and, in the worst cases it can cause skin cancer. Yet a hint of a tan does make us look and feel good. So this is where fake wins over real every time.

Fake tan is something you can do throughout the year and, if applied correctly can have beautiful, realistic results. A good fake tan can make your limbs look instantly longer. It's also great camouflage for that scourge of female flesh – cellulite.

How to do it

* Start with a shower or a bath where you exfoliate by either body brushing or using a body scrub.

* Once out of the bath apply a non-greasy moisturiser all over your body, paying particular attention to areas such as heels, knees and elbows – any areas where your skin is a little dry.

* It is always best to apply your fake tan using gloves, or your bronzed palms will give away the fact that your tan is fake and not the result of a jet-setting lifestyle.

* Apply small amounts – a little goes a long way – and start from your feet and work up. Allow at least five minutes before dressing.

* To maintain your healthy glow, apply twice a week.

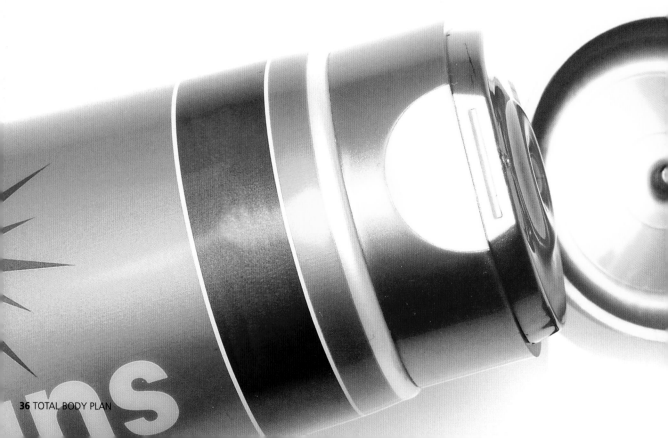

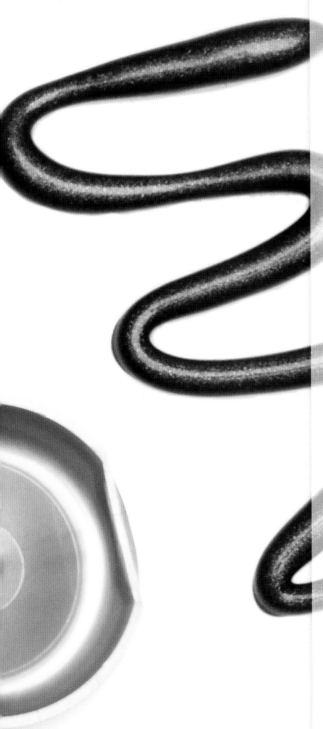

Q&A

YOUR QUESTIONS ANSWERED

Q I always have an energy crash around 4pm. I have a nap but then feel tired for the rest of the day. How can I shrug off this feeling?

A: The best and only way for you to restore your energy is with exercise. It takes just a little motivation to get going, but once you're a couple of minutes into it you will feel wide awake. As you get fitter, your energy levels will stay higher throughout the day.

Q Every time in the past when I have tried to lose weight I ended up putting more on. Will the same happen with this plan?

A: No. The chances are that your previous attempts at weight loss put an unreasonable strain on your lifestyle, so you didn't keep it up and quickly regained any weight you'd lost. This programme is designed to fit in easily with any lifestyle. It is easy to follow, safe and realistic. You will be eating sensibly, which will ensure you lose body fat as opposed to muscle, and the regular exercise will help you to tone muscles and increase the amount of calories you burn naturally on a daily basis.

Best of all, because the programme doesn't require lots of free time or access to fancy gyms, it will not interfere with your normal routine, so you are less likely to give up half way through.

Q How can I get myself motivated if I am having an off day?

A: For me, music is one of the best motivators there is. Find an upbeat song that you like, play it loud and do just one of your exercises to some fast tunes. The great thing is that the minute you start exercising you instantly feel better. Exercise encourages your body to produce feel-good hormones. Pretty soon you'll want to complete your whole workout.

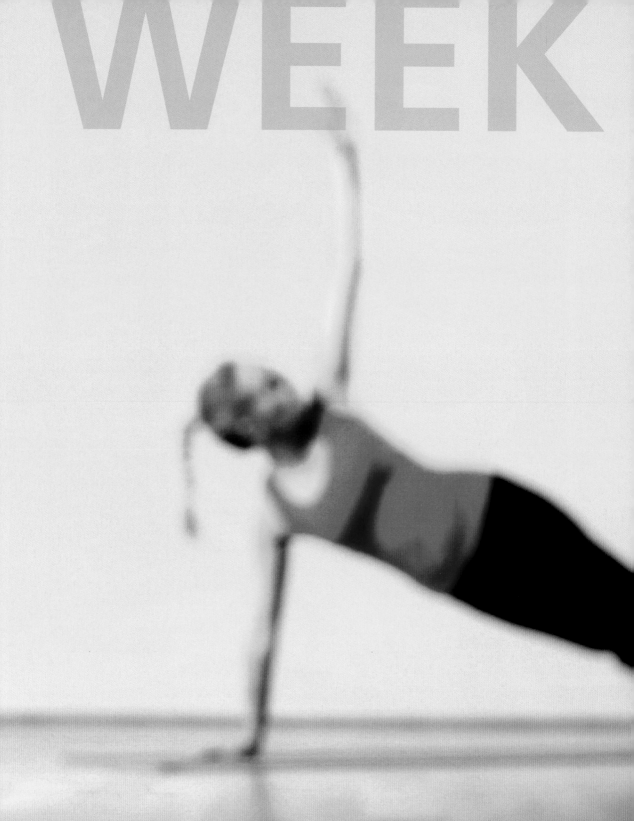

TWO

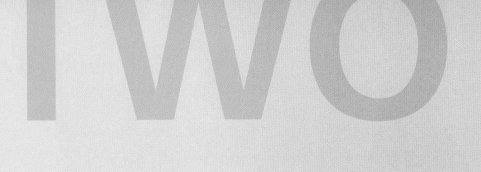

'If you could buy fitness in a jar, we would all be fit'

the plan...

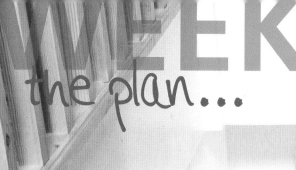

Monday 15-minute stair sculpt see opposite

Tuesday 1 x home circuit see p42

Wednesday 15-minute stair sculpt

Thursday 1 x home circuit

Friday 15-minute stair sculpt

Saturday 2 x home circuits

Sunday Rest

TOP TIP

To work you legs, butt and improve your balance, take two stairs at a time whenever you are using the stairs. Avoid holding the banisters to further improve your balance

Aerobic
15-minute stair sculpt

In Week Two this easy to follow stair sculpt aerobic workout will leave you feeling more energetic, it'll burn calories and give you tone all over. By going to your 'home gym', ie your staircase, you'll work deep into the muscles of your lower body. Alongside this, the exercises on the following pages will tone your waist and upper body. Even if you are tight on time, you should still be able to squeeze this one in three times a week.

Get the most out of it

* When you run upstairs, ensure your posture is good, back upright and shoulders relaxed.

* Lift your knees as you go up and stay on the balls of your feet. Swing your arms in time with your feet and keep the whole movement rhythmical. Always ensure you foot is placed fully on the stair.

* For the side squat, simply stand side-on to the bottom stair, keeping one foot firmly on the ground and the other on the first step. Both feet should be facing forwards at about shoulder-width apart. Place your hands on your hips, slowly bend through your knees and stick your bottom out as if you are about to sit on a chair. Hold for a second then slowly push back up.

Time (mins)	Exercise	Perceived rate of exertion
0–2	Warm up by walking up and down the stairs	4
2–4	Walk briskly up the stairs, repeatedly bringing your arms over your head and back down	5
4–5	Run up and down the stairs	6
5–6	Now march up, taking two stairs at a time. Step normally on the way back down	5
6–8	Side squat, one minute on each leg. See left for details	5
8–9	Now march up, taking two stairs at a time. Step normally on the way back down	5
9–10	Run up and down the stairs	6
10–11	Now place both your hands behind your head and march up and down the stairs	5
11–13	Side squat, one minute on each leg. See left for details	5
13–14	Run up and down the stairs	6
14–15	Cool down by walking up and down the stairs	4

Home circuits
Just ten minutes

Warm up for two to three minutes (see p18), then perform the five exercises in order. Do each for one minute before moving straight on to the next with no rest in between. Once you've finished spend two minutes doing some stretching (see p19)

Start here →

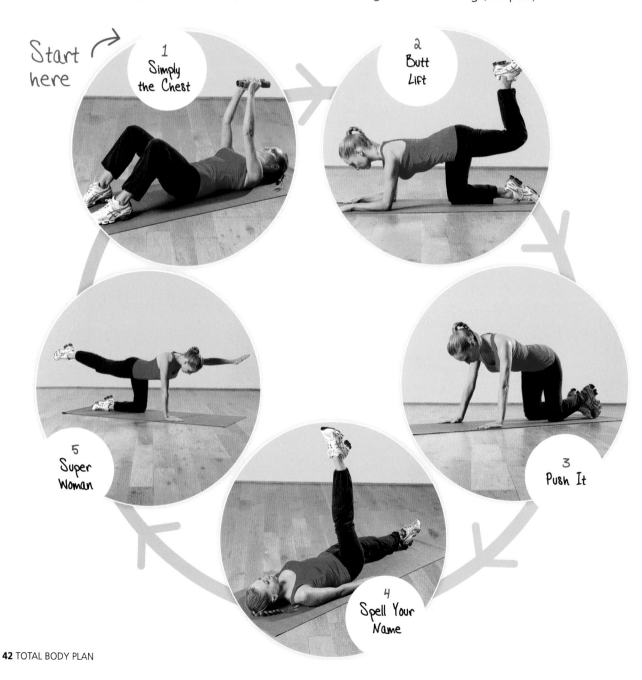

1 Simply the Chest

2 Butt Lift

3 Push It

4 Spell Your Name

5 Super Woman

Exercise one

Simply the Chest

What it does
This floor exercise specifically targets your bust, helping to improve muscle tone and prevent your breasts from sagging over time.

How to do it
Lie on your back on your mat, with knees bent and feet flat on the floor.

Start with a weight or water bottle in each hand and your arms extended over you chest with palms facing each other. Your elbows should not lock. Slowly lower your arms out to the sides without letting them rest on the floor. Return to the start and repeat. Ensure you keep your shoulders still throughout.

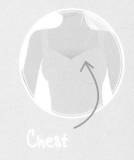

Chest

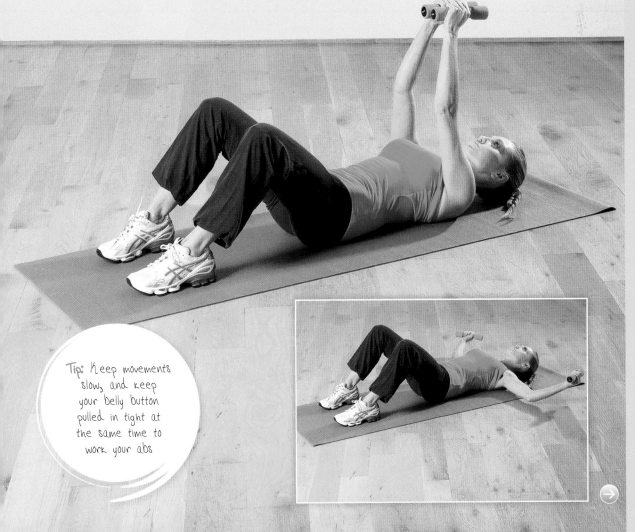

Tip: Keep movements slow, and keep your belly button pulled in tight at the same time to work your abs

43

Exercise two

Butt Lift

What it does
This easy floor exercise works on toning and lifting the glutes, thus giving you a pert derrière, at the same time working the backs of your upper thighs.

How to do it
Kneel on all fours on your mat, with your forearms and palms flat on the floor. Your back should be straight and slightly below horizontal. Lift your left knee off the floor and raise your heel to the ceiling, then lower the knee and cross it behind your right leg, before returning to the start. Continue with the left leg for 30 seconds then switch to the right for a further 30 seconds.

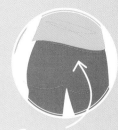

Bottom

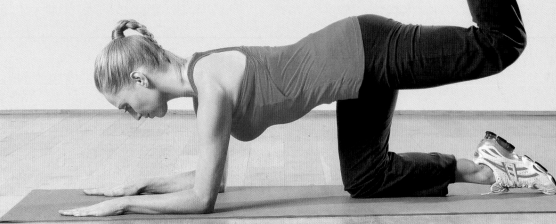

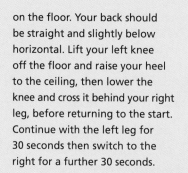

Tip: Work on keeping your belly button pulled up to the spine throughout as this will support your back and work your abs at the same time

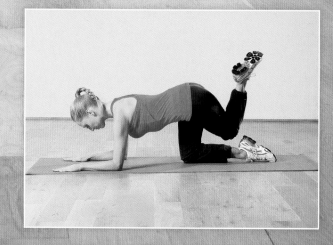

Exercise three

Push It

What it does

This is a great way of toning up your arms and adding volume to your chest. It will give shape to your triceps – the rear upper arms – and make your cleavage appear fuller.

How to do it

Kneel on all fours, hands just ahead of your shoulders, arms straight. Your body should form a straight line from head to hips. Keeping your tummy pulled in, bend your elbows to lower your body until your chest is about three inches from the floor, then push back up to the start. Repeat for one minute.

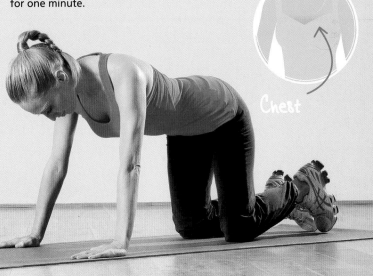

Triceps

Chest

Tip: To make this more challenging push your hips forward and create a straight line from your knees to your hips

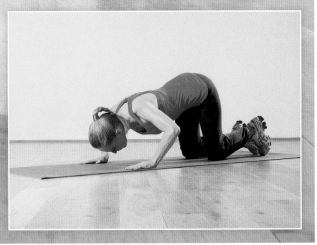

Exercise four

Spell Your Name

What it does

This fun exercise is great for toning your thighs and giving the abs a workout at the same time.

How to do it

Lie on your mat with your arms by your sides and your palms facing down. Raise your right leg, keeping it straight and pointing the toes as if reaching towards the ceiling. Rotate your leg slightly outward, inhale, and trace the first letter of your name on the ceiling with your toes. Move the whole leg but keep your hips still by pulling your belly button in tight to your spine. Concentrate on not lifting your left hip off the floor. Continue to draw each letter of your name. Do this for 30 seconds then repeat with your left leg.

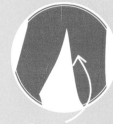

Thighs

Abs

Tip: Keep this slow and controlled

Exercise five

Super Woman

What it does

This clever exercise works all your abdominal muscles as you engage them to help keep your balance. It's also very good for helping to strengthen your lower back.

How to do it

Kneel on all fours on your mat, hands directly under shoulders and knees directly under hips. Take a deep breath and, as you slowly exhale, tighten your stomach and simultaneously straighten your left arm and your right leg, bringing your foot to hip height and your hand to shoulder height. There should be a line running from foot to hip, through your torso to your hand. Keep the abs tight and be sure not to rotate your hips. Hold for a five count then slowly return to the start. Repeat with the opposite arm and leg and continue for one minute.

Abs

Lower back

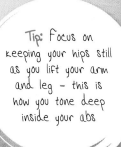

Tip: Focus on keeping your hips still as you lift your arm and leg – this is how you tone deep inside your abs

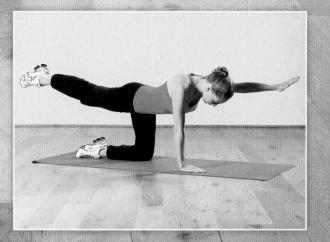

tuck in...

Monday	Tuesday

Breakfast
Anti-cellulite smoothie
(see p53)

Mid-morning snack
Carrot and cucumber
sticks with a little low-fat
cottage cheese

Lunch
Wholemeal pitta stuffed
with slices of lean turkey,
salad, tomatoes and a
small amount of low-fat
grated cheese

Mid-afternoon snack
3 ham slices wrapped
around asparagus spears

Dinner
Steamed cod with steamed
mangetouts, baby carrots
and spinach

Breakfast
Make you own cereal by
adding chopped dried fruit,
raisins and seeds to a good
handful of porridge oats

Mid-morning snack
2 oatcakes with small
slices of cheese

Lunch
Tin of soup with a toasted
pitta, banana

Mid-afternoon snack
Hard-boiled egg with
raw carrots

Dinner
Either grilled chicken
breast or Quorn fillet,
served with mashed sweet
potato and sweetcorn

Wednesday

Breakfast
Bowl of cereal with sliced banana

Mid-morning snack
Bunch of grapes and small slice of cheese

Lunch
Chicken salad with avocado

Mid-afternoon snack
Handful of nuts and dried fruit

Dinner
Prawn and vegetable stir-fry

Thursday

Breakfast
2 slices of wholemeal toast with peanut butter or a poached egg

Mid-morning snack
150g pot of low-fat yoghurt

Lunch
Small jacket potato filled with low-fat cottage cheese and chopped peppers

Mid-afternoon snack
Small cup of homemade popcorn

Dinner
Grilled turkey breast with steamed spinach and mangetouts, served with brown rice

Wait for pudding
If you still feel hungry after a meal, wait 20 minutes before having pudding. It takes that long for the signal to get from your stomach to your brain that you're already full

continued...

Friday	Saturday	Sunday

Breakfast
Bowl of mixed fruit salad with natural live yoghurt and 2tsp of porridge oats

Mid-morning snack
Handful of nuts and raisins

Lunch
Homemade vegetable soup with a toasted pitta

Mid-afternoon snack
Oatcakes with tbsp of cottage cheese and cherry tomatoes

Dinner
Grilled turkey breast with stir-fried vegetables

Breakfast
Omelette made with whites of two eggs and peppers and onions

Mid-morning snack
Small cup of homemade popcorn

Lunch
Mixed bean salad: tbsp each of red kidney beans, chickpeas and cannellini beans mixed with sweetcorn and tomatoes, wholemeal pitta

Mid-afternoon snack
Toasted crumpet with drizzle of honey

Dinner
Grilled cod drizzled with lemon butter, served with grilled tomatoes, peppers and courgettes

Breakfast
Grilled lean bacon, grilled tomatoes, mushrooms and slice of wholemeal toast

Mid-morning snack
Banana with handful of raisins

Lunch
Small jacket potato with tuna and spring onions

Mid-afternoon snack
150g pot of low-fat yoghurt

Dinner
Grilled chicken breast with mashed sweet potato and minted peas

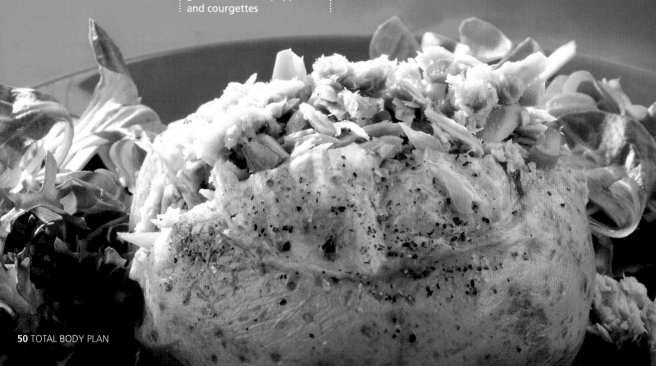

Shopping list

Wholemeal pittas and bread
Brown rice
Crumpets, for toasting
Oatcakes
Popcorn
Pomegranate juice
Low-fat milk, yoghurts, cottage cheese, hard cheese
Soya milk
Peanut butter
Honey
Cereal, porridge oats
Mixed nuts and seeds
Ground flaxseed
Raisins, mixed dried fruit
Fruit/veg: apples, asparagus, avocados, bananas, carrots, cherry
tomatoes, courgettes, cucumber, grapes, jacket potatoes,
lemons, leeks, mangetouts, mixed berries, mushrooms, onions,
oranges, peas, peppers, salad leaves, spinach, spring onions,
sweetcorn, sweet potatoes, tomatoes
Turkey slices (cooked)
Chicken slices (cooked)
Ham slices (cooked)
Tins of tuna, soup, chickpeas, cannellini beans, red kidney beans
Turkey breasts
Chicken breasts
Lean bacon
Cod
Prawns
Eggs

Food facts
The truth about cellulite

Cellulite, which is often referred to as the orange-peel effect, creeps up on women of all shapes and sizes, from the underweight to the overweight. The reason is simple: we all have fat cells.

Cellulite is nothing more than fat. As women, our fat cells are shaped differently to men's – ours run horizontally and men's run diagonally. When a woman's fats cells become enlarged – due to her eating the wrong foods and not doing regular exercise – they squish upwards and show through her skin. This is what causes the dimply effect known as cellulite.

So, if we choose to have an unhealthy lifestyle that consists of doing no exercise and eating a diet of processed foods high in fat, sugar and salt, and if we drink more coffee and alcohol than we should, then we are sending an open invitation to the dreaded cellulite to move in and settle down on hotspots such as our thighs, bottoms, tummies and arms.

The best way to reduce the appearance of cellulite is a combination of regular exercise, good nutrition, drinking plenty of water and body brushing (see page 54).

The great thing about all of these things is that, not only will they help reduce your cellulite, they will also tone you up, improve your wellbeing, give you loads of energy and leave you radiant with health and vitality.

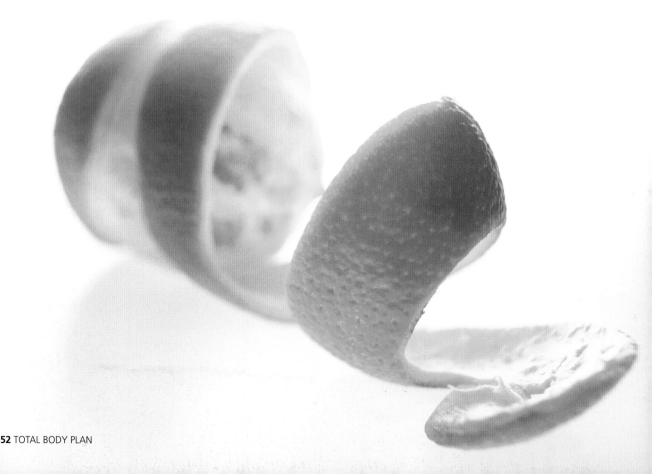

Blend it
Anti-cellulite smoothie

This is quick and simple to make, and it's packed full of metabolism-boosting fruit and plenty of water, as well as fibrous ingredients to help banish orange-peel thighs

Chuck it all in a blender, whiz it and drink it

Ingredients

* 2 tablespoons of unsweetened pomegranate juice
* 3 tablespoons of soya milk
* Handful of blueberries
* 2 tablespoons of goji berries
* 2 tablespoons of ground flaxseed
* 5-6 ice cubes

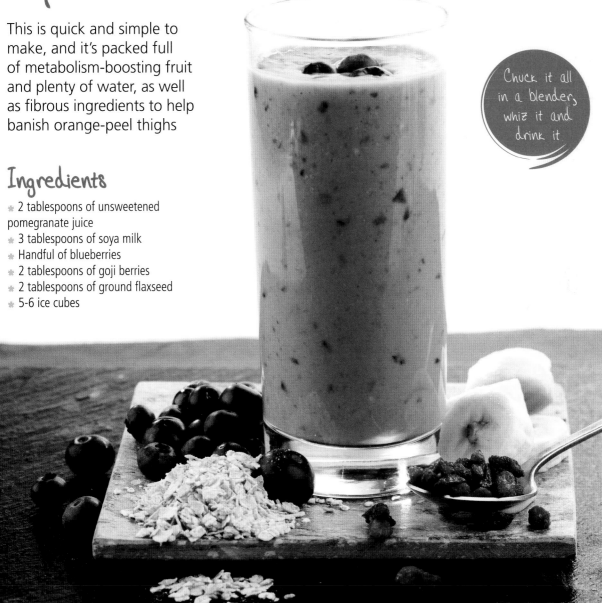

Look great
Body brushing

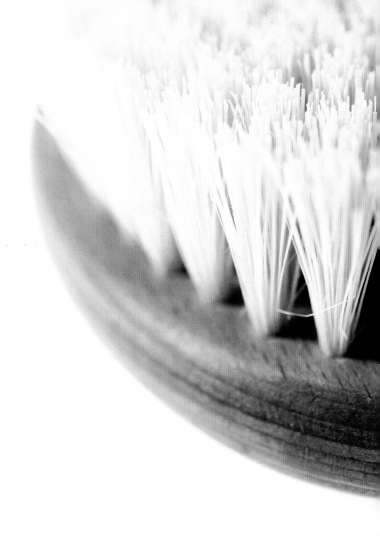

Body brushing, also known as skin brushing, is a very important part of your skincare routine and ideally should be done at least twice a week. It helps to reduce cellulite by breaking down fatty deposits, and it aids in the lymphatic drainage and detoxification processes. It will also remove any dead skin cells, instantly making your skin look younger as well as encouraging your cells to regenerate.

Body brushes are made with natural bristles, can be found in any good chemist and are a very worthwhile investment. This is a great habit to get into – it takes less that three minutes.

How to do it

* After you have rinsed off in the bath or shower, take the brush and begin with the sole of your right foot. Use firm, rhythmic strokes to cover the sole several times. Next, brush the top of your foot, towards your ankle. Then go on to your lower leg, making sure you cover the whole surface. Finish off on your thigh, then do the other leg. Always brush in an upward direction, towards the heart.

* Next, brush your right arm. Start with the palm of your hand, then move on to the back of your hand. Next brush from your wrist up to your elbow. Brush your upper arm, working from your elbow towards your shoulder, again covering the whole surface. Then, very gently, brush your abdomen, using a circular motion, always in a clockwise direction. Cover the area several times but with less pressure than on your arms and legs. Then finish off with the chest area, the skin is a lot more sensitive here so be gentle. Finish off by applying moisturiser to your entire body – your skin will now feel incredible. Repeat two to three times a week.

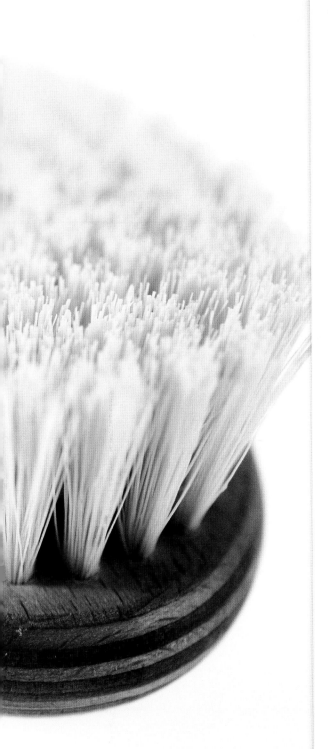

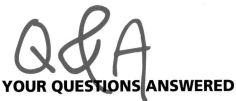

YOUR QUESTIONS ANSWERED

 Why do my muscles ache after exercise?

A: This is a great question because it is relevant to everyone from the top athlete to the first-time exerciser. Simply put, every time we exercise we put strain on our muscles, which causes tiny tears in the muscle structure. But the human body is amazing – the muscles then repair the tears, becoming stronger in the process. Warming down and stretching after your workout helps the muscles to repair themselves, as well as flushing out toxins, which both reduce that next-day soreness.

 Should I exercise on an empty stomach?

A: No, you should never exercise on an empty stomach. If you exercise early in the morning, a banana and small glass of milk will give you energy. If you work out a bit later in the day, aim to have a snack 30 minutes before you exercise.

 Does muscle weigh less than fat?

A: Muscle is more dense than fat, so it weighs more than the same volume of fat. Two people can be the same height and have the same measurements, but the person who has more fat will weigh less than the person who has more muscle. This is why I am a big fan of the tape measure as opposed to the scales.

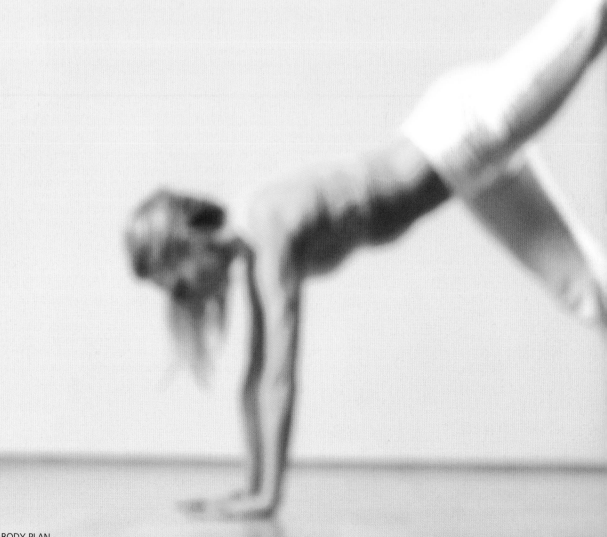

WEEK

'A strong outside strengthens the inside'

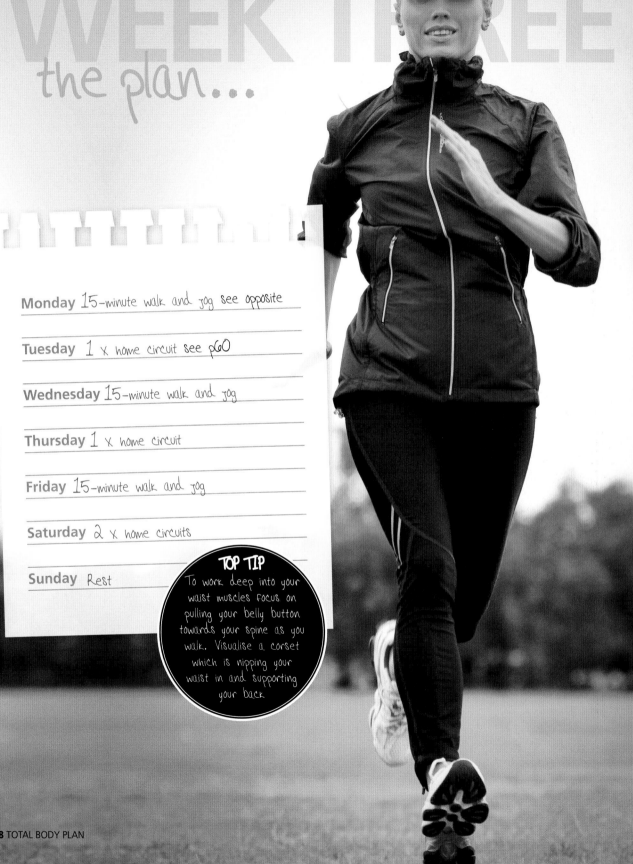

the plan...

Monday 15-minute walk and jog see opposite

Tuesday 1 x home circuit see p60

Wednesday 15-minute walk and jog

Thursday 1 x home circuit

Friday 15-minute walk and jog

Saturday 2 x home circuits

Sunday Rest

TOP TIP

To work deep into your waist muscles focus on pulling your belly button towards your spine as you walk. Visualise a corset which is nipping your waist in and supporting your back

Aerobic
15-minute walk and jog

In Week Three your aerobic workout will combine power walking and gentle running. This will burn off any excess weight, banish love handles and sculpt your glutes and abs in no time at all. It's also a great way to improve your overall fitness.

Walk before you run

* As mentioned on page 23, always walk with good posture. Keep your shoulders, hips and ankles in a vertical line, your shoulders relaxed, and bend your elbows to about 90°.
* As you walk keep your knees soft.
* Always land on your heel and push off from the front of your foot.
* When jogging and running try to keep your stride low to the ground and focus on quick turnover.
* Too much up-and-down movement is hard on your lower body – the higher you lift yourself off the ground, the greater the shock you have to absorb when landing and the faster your legs will fatigue.

Time (mins)	Exercise	Perceived rate of exertion
0–2	Gentle walk for a warm-up	3–4
2–4	Brisk walk, keeping abs pulled in	5
4–5	Gentle jog	5
5–6	Run	6
6–8	Gentle jog	5
8–10	Brisk walk, keeping abs pulled in	5
10–11	Gentle jog	5
11–12	Run	6
12–13	Gentle jog	5
13–14	Brisk walk, keeping abs pulled in	5
14–15	Cool down by slowly reducing your walking pace	4

Home circuits
Just ten minutes

Warm up for two to three minutes (see p18), then perform the five exercises in order. Do each for one minute before moving straight on to the next with no rest in between. Once you've finished spend two minutes doing some stretching (see p19)

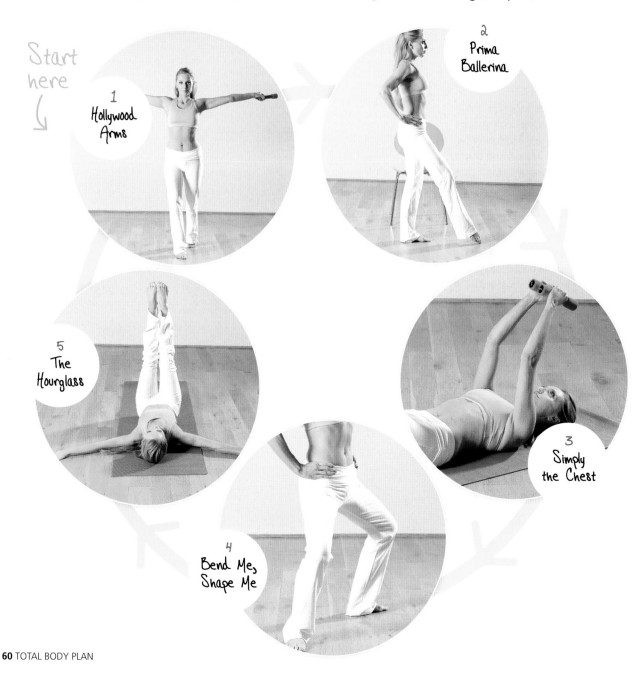

Start here

1 Hollywood Arms

2 Prima Ballerina

3 Simply the Chest

4 Bend Me, Shape Me

5 The Hourglass

Exercise one

Hollywood Arms

What it does

This simple exercise feels very easy at first – you could be fooled into thinking you could do it for hours. But trust me, it's not long before you start to feel those muscles working. In no time you'll have beautiful, slender arms – just like the movie stars.

How to do it

Stand with good posture, one foot ahead of the other, both feet pointing forward and knees slightly bent. Hold your arms at shoulder height, palms facing down, fingers pointed. Slowly start to make small circles and keep these going anti-clockwise for 30 seconds before switching to clockwise for 30 seconds.

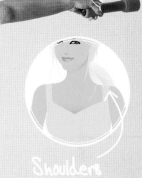

Shoulders

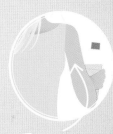

Triceps

Tip: Work your abs by pulling them in tight. As you become fitter you can make this more challenging by holding water bottles or weights

61

Exercise two

Prima Ballerina

What it does

This exercise is used by dancers, as it improves posture and tones the thighs, buttocks and abdominals. The rotation improves hip mobility and tones the hip area, while the circular motion firms and lifts the buttocks. Again, this elegant routine will also work your abs if you keep them tucked in.

How to do it

Standing with good posture, place your weight on your left leg and extend your right leg in front of you. Use the back of a chair to maintain balance. Squeeze in your right buttock and slowly sweep your right leg to the side, keeping the abs pulled in. Maintaining the squeeze, now circle the leg behind you. Breathing evenly throughout, perform this exercise for 30 seconds with either leg.

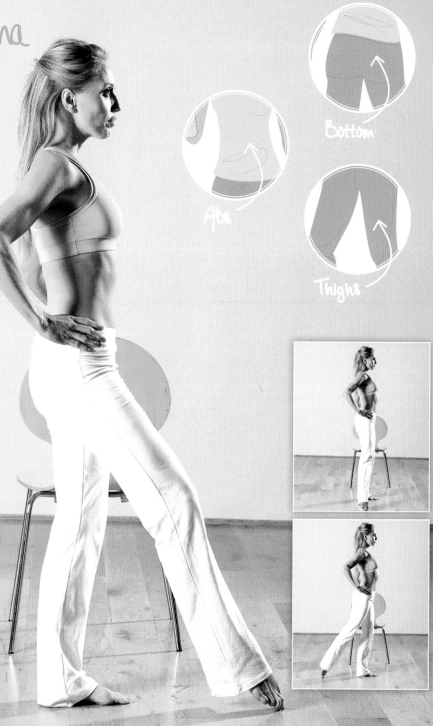

Abs

Bottom

Thighs

Tip: Focus on creating a big circle with the moving leg as this will really help to tone and lift the bottom

Exercise three
Simply the Chest

What it does

As we get older the muscles that support the bust lengthen, which results in the bust becoming less firm. This easy exercise will help to reverse this.

How to do it

Lie on your back, knees bent and feet flat on the floor, with your arms extended to the ceiling, elbows slightly bent. Be sure to hold your weights or water bottles above your chest and not your face. Lower your arms until your elbows almost touch the floor. Hold for a second then slowly return to the start position. Repeat for one minute.

Chest

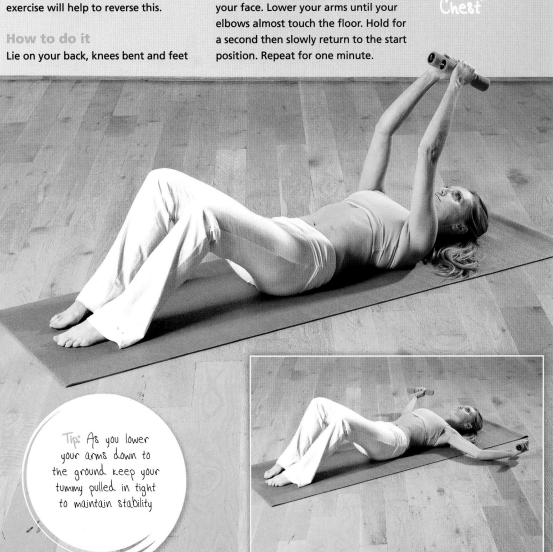

Tip: As you lower your arms down to the ground keep your tummy pulled in tight to maintain stability

Exercise four

Bend Me, Shape Me

What it does

You get to tone your hips, thighs, bottom and abs all at once using this ballet-inspired move.

How to do it

Stand with your feet slightly wider than shoulder-width apart, toes pointing out, hands on hips. Slowly bend your knees and lower yourself into a squat, making sure you keep your upper body straight. Hold for a second, then come back up to the start position. Repeat for one minute.

Tip: Focus on squeezing your bottom in tight on the way down and coming back up

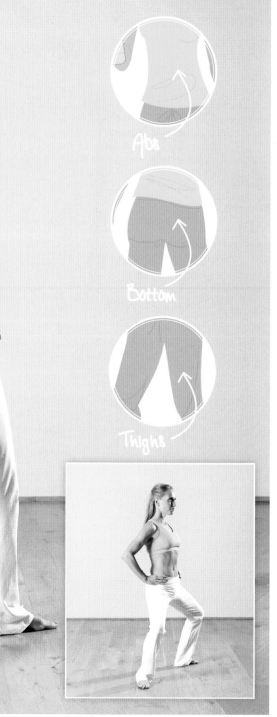

Abs

Bottom

Thighs

Exercise five

The Hourglass

What it does

By drawing in the oblique muscles that shape your waist, this will give you that feminine hourglass shape.

How to do it

Lie on your back, arms out in line with shoulders, palms on the floor. Raise both your legs and, keeping them pressed tightly together, point the toes so that your legs are fully extended directly over your hips. Engage your abdominal muscles by pulling your belly button in tight to your spine, then slowly sway your legs a few inches to the left. Hold, then return them to the centre, before slowly swaying to the right. Repeat for one minute, making sure your lower back stays on the floor throughout.

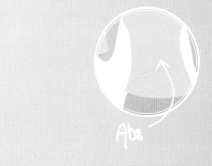

Abs

Tip: As your abdominals become stronger you can make the movement slightly bigger

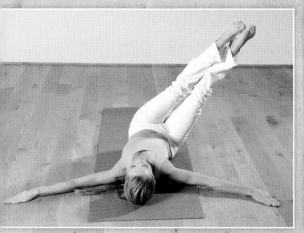

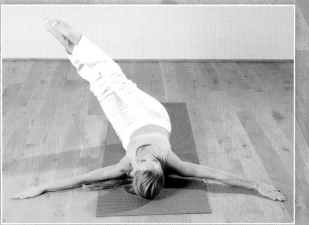

MEAL PLAN

tuck in...

Monday	Tuesday

Breakfast
Omelette made with
2 egg whites and sliced
red and green peppers

Mid-morning snack
150g pot of low-fat yoghurt

Lunch
Beetroot and goat's cheese
salad on spinach leaves

Mid-afternoon snack
3 pieces of fruit

Dinner
Grilled tuna steak with
pineapple chilli relish,
served with salad

Breakfast
Porridge with berries

Mid-morning snack
Sliced avocado and
cherry tomatoes

Lunch
Wholemeal pitta stuffed
with low-fat cottage cheese
and red onion

Mid-afternoon snack
Anti-wrinkle smoothie
(see p71)

Dinner
Wholemeal spaghetti with
lean turkey mince

Don't be fooled by labels

'90% fat free!' may sound healthy, but it still means that your food has 10% fat, which is a lot. Also 'reduced fat' can mean increased sugar, which is just as fattening

Wednesday

Breakfast
2 slices of wholemeal toast with a small tin of plum tomatoes

Mid-morning snack
Handful of homemade popcorn

Lunch
Wholegrain bagel with tuna and sweetcorn

Mid-afternoon snack
Sugar-free protein bar

Dinner
Wholemeal spaghetti with lean steak mince

Thursday

Breakfast
Porridge with a sprinkling of berries and seeds

Mid-morning snack
Rice cake with avocado

Lunch
Bowl of carrot soup with added butter beans

Mid-afternoon snack
Hard-boiled egg with raw carrots

Dinner
Lean beef steak with green beans and a small jacket potato

Friday	Saturday	Sunday

Breakfast
Anti-wrinkle smoothie
(see p71)

Mid-morning snack
2 Ryvitas with ham slices
and cucumber

Lunch
Wholemeal wrap with
avocado, tomato and
low-fat mozzarella

Mid-afternoon snack
Handful of nuts and raisins

Dinner
Poached salmon with leeks
and green vegetables

Breakfast
Crêpes with fresh fruit

Mid-morning snack
2 oatcakes topped
with avocado

Lunch
Omelette made with 2 egg
whites, herbs and spinach

Mid-afternoon snack
Sliced cucumber, carrots and
peppers with hummus dip

Dinner
Grilled chicken with
wholemeal penne pasta in
a tomato-based sauce

Breakfast
Scrambled egg with
smoked salmon

Mid-morning snack
Banana and a handful
of nuts

Lunch
Chicken Caesar salad

Mid-afternoon snack
1 toasted crumpet with
a drizzle of honey

Dinner
Stir-fried beef with butternut
squash and green beans

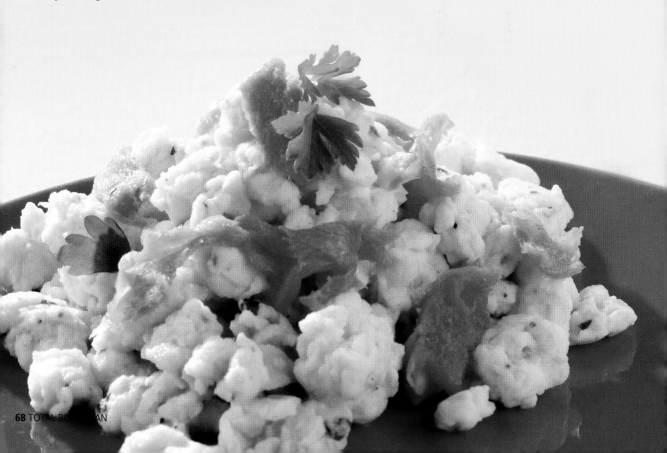

Shopping list

Wholemeal bagels, bread, penne pasta, pittas, spaghetti, wraps
Crêpes
Crumpets, for toasting
Low-fat yoghurts, cottage cheese, mozzarella, hard cheese
hummus, goats cheese
Honey
Ryvita
Rice cakes
Porridge oats
Popcorn
Nuts and raisins
Mixed seeds
Fruit/veg: apples, avocados, bananas, beetroot, butternut squash,
carrots, cherry toms, cucumber, frozen berries, green beans, jacket
potatoes, kiwi fruits, leeks, melon, oranges, peppers, red onion,
salad leaves, spinach, strawberries, sweetcorn, sweet potatoes, tomatoes
Ham slices (cooked)
Lean beef steak
Chicken breasts
Salmon fillets
Tuna steak
Lean steak mince, lean turkey mince
Smoked salmon
Tins of tuna, carrot soup, plum tomatoes, butter beans
Eggs
Pineapple chilli relish
Caesar salad dressing
Soy sauce
Fresh ginger
Sugar-free protein bar

Fit facts
Turn back the clock

You are never too old to start looking younger. And lifestyle is the key. Eating the right foods, doing the right exercise and having the right attitude will make you look – and feel – younger.

Exercise is a great way to feel the years falling away. This doesn't mean spending hours in a gym or running marathons. It means making exercise part of your routine. Women today often describe themselves as 'time poor': we have to juggle family, work and home. This is why I designed the workouts

in this book so that you can do them at home and easily make them part of your busy day.

The other great news is that the fitter you get the more energy you have. You'll enjoy working out more and more. As well as the benefits of making you feel strong and good about yourself, exercise increases the amount of oxygen in your blood, which gives you a glowing complexion and improves your skin, hair and nails – all of which take years off.

So, if you're after a magical way to recover your youth, choose the trainers over Botox.

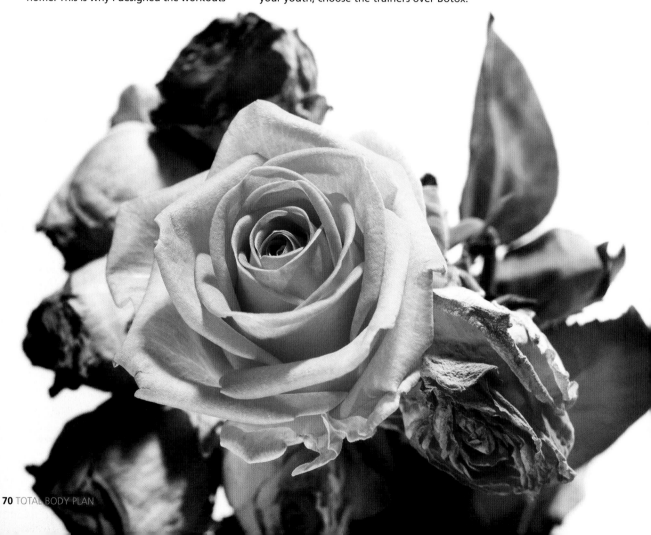

Blend it
Anti-wrinkle smoothie

This tasty smoothie is packed full of fruits that are rich in vitamin C. Vitamin C is responsible for the production of collagen, which keeps skin plumped up and prevents wrinkles. Not only does it work wonders for your skin, it's also a great way to strengthen your immune system, bones and joints.

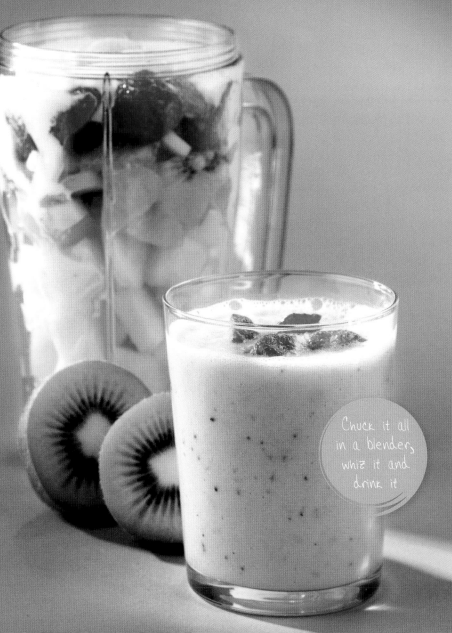

Chuck it all in a blender, whiz it and drink it

Ingredients

* Chopped kiwi fruit
* Handful of strawberries
* Half a melon
* Orange
* Low-fat natural yoghurt
* 1cm slice of fresh ginger

Look great
Anti-ageing face mask

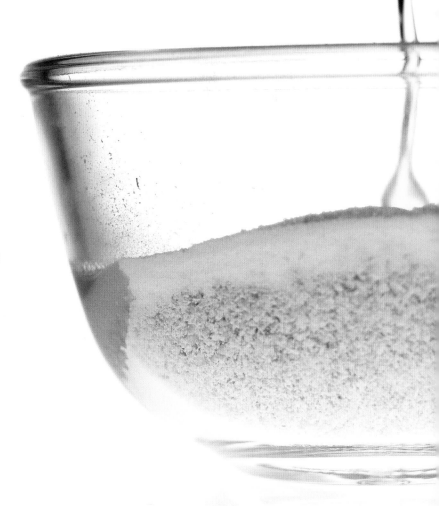

Take years off your face with no mess, no needles and no surgery. This anti-ageing face mask will have you radiating health and wellbeing. It's simple to make and can be applied once a week. It'll improve your circulation and remove any dead skin cells, leaving you with a glowing complexion.

What you need

* **Almond oil for fair skin**

* **Olive oil for dark skin**

* **Jojoba for sensitive skin**

* **Fine oatmeal or table salt**

How to do it

* Simply put eight drops of the oil that's right for your skin type into the palm of your hand and apply all over your face.

* Then apply your exfoliate – either your oatmeal or salt mixed with several drops of your oil and made into a paste. Using the pads of your fingers, rub it in evenly all over your face and neck in a light action.

* Don't forget to rub a little of the mixture into your lips to plump them up. Leave on for a few minutes then rinse off the mixture with warm water. To finish off apply your normal moisturiser.

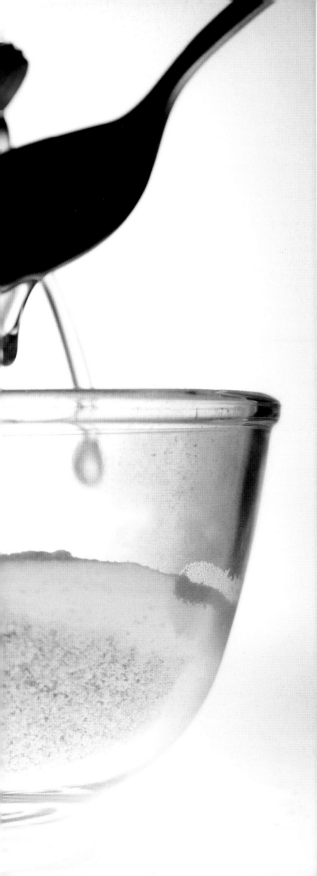

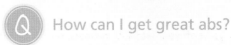

YOUR QUESTIONS ANSWERED

Q How can I get great abs?

A: It takes three things to have amazing abdominals: aerobic exercise, circuits and healthy eating. This programme works on all three, so stick to it and you'll be working towards having that super-toned tummy.

Q I want to lose a stone in weight. How soon can I start to expect to see results and how long will it take?

A: If you exercise at least three times a week, after three weeks you should notice a huge difference. My clients lose 1–1.5kg per week, which is as much as you should lose on a weekly basis to guarantee you don't then pile it all back on again – and more. The great thing with exercise is that each time you work out you will feel energised and glowing. So if you eat sensibly and train properly, you could lose a stone within five weeks.

Q Will exercise help to improve my posture?

A: Absolutely. Exercise is a great way to realign your body, as it strengthens your skeletal muscles and makes your bones stronger. You will naturally find that your posture improves throughout this programme.

WEEK

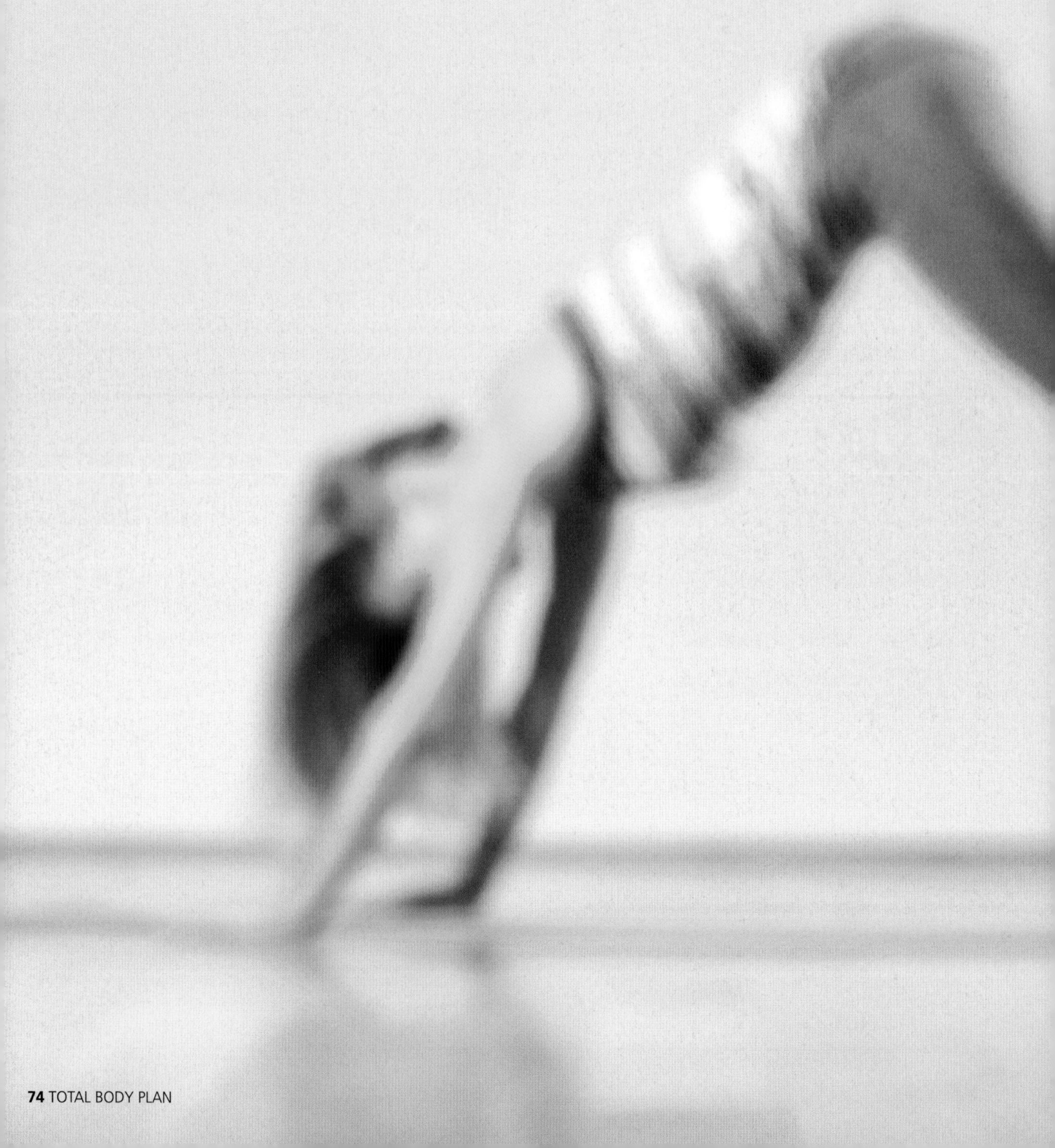

FOUR

'If you don't focus on your butt, no one else will'

the plan...

Monday *15*-minute boot camp see opposite

Tuesday *1* x home circuit see p78

Wednesday *15*-minute boot camp

Thursday *1* x home circuit

Friday *15*-minute boot camp

Saturday *2* x home circuits

Sunday Rest

TOP TIP

When doing high-impact moves (when both feet are off the floor at the same time) land as lightly as you can on your feet and keep your knees soft as this reduces the impact on your joints

Aerobic
15-minute boot camp

Week Four is your very own boot camp. This specially designed workout will have you as fit as GI Jane. You need no equipment and it can be done indoors or outdoors. Each exercise gets your heart rate up and your body burning calories.

Magnificent seven
Your boot camp consists of seven exercises: marching and jogging on the spot, as well as these:

❋ Star jumps
Jump up, opening your legs wide and throwing your arms out, creating a star shape while in the air.

❋ Jumps from side to side
Bend your knees and lean slightly forwards from your waist, jump right, landing with your knees slightly bent, pause, then jump to the left.

❋ Alternating lunges
Stand with feet hip-width apart, pointing forward, hands on hips. Take a large step forward with either leg, bend your knees, keeping your upper body straight, then push through the heel in front to bring yourself back. Then lead with the other leg.

❋ Knee lifts
Start with feet hip-width apart, abs pulled in tight. Lift one knee to hip height, lower, then switch knees.

❋ Step-ups
March on and off the bottom step.

Time (mins)	Exercise	Perceived rate of exertion
0–1	March on the spot	3–4
1–2	Jumps from side to side	5
2–3	Alternate lunges	5
3–4	Jog on the spot	6
4–5	Star jumps	5
5–6	Alternate knee lifts	5
6–7	Step-ups on bottom stair	5
7–8	Jumps from side to side	6
8–9	Alternate lunges	5
9–10	Jog on the spot	6
10–11	Star jumps	5
11–12	Alternate knee lifts	5
12–13	Step-ups on bottom stair	5
13–14	Jumps from side to side	5
14–15	March on spot to cool down	4

77

Home circuits
Just ten minutes

Warm up for two to three minutes (see p18), then perform the five exercises in order. Do each for one minute before moving straight on to the next with no rest in between. Once you've finished spend two minutes doing some stretching (see p19)

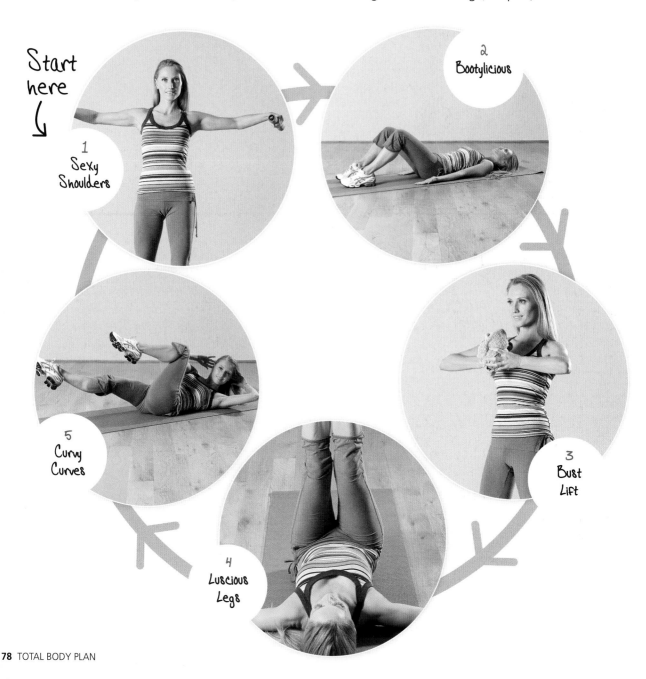

Start here ↳

1 Sexy Shoulders

2 Bootylicious

3 Bust Lift

4 Luscious Legs

5 Curvy Curves

Exercise one

Sexy Shoulders

What it does

This exercise will help to define your shoulders and triceps. It's also good for improving flexibility in your shoulder joints and it'll give you good posture.

How to do it

Stand with your feet shoulder-width apart and your knees slightly bent. Hold your hand weights or water bottles at your sides at thigh level. Slowly lift the weights out to the sides to shoulder level, keeping your elbows slightly bent. Keep your shoulders down and relaxed as you lift. If you find you're shrugging your shoulders up toward your ears, your weights may be too heavy. Slowly lower the weights back to your sides. Do this for one minute.

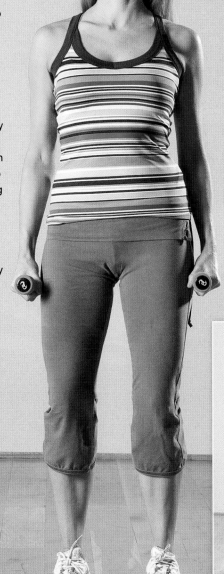

Tip: It's important to keep a slight bend in the arms as you lift. Imagine you're holding a teacup in each hand and you're pouring water from them. This helps keep the arms soft

Shoulders

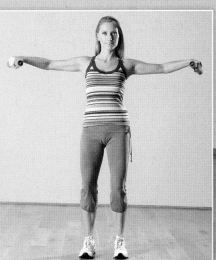

Exercise two

Bootylicious

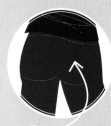

Bum

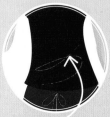

Abs

What it does

This is the perfect exercise to get you that great bum you've always wanted – or to keep the one you've got. It not only tones those glutes, it'll also rev up your metabolism so that you'll be burning off extra calories throughout the day.

How to do it

Lie face up with your arms at your sides, knees bent and feet flat on the floor. Lift your hips toward the ceiling, squeezing your bottom muscles tight. Hold this position for two seconds, then lower yourself back down. Repeat for one minute.

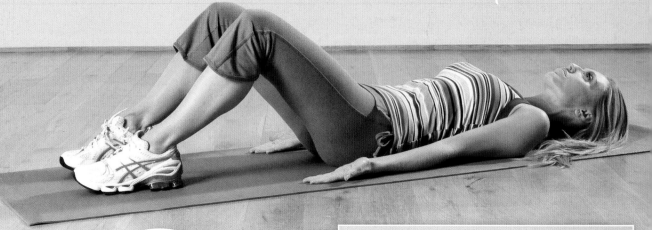

Tip: As you lift your bottom off the floor keep your abdominals pulled in tight. This will protect your back and work your abs

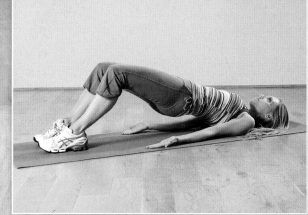

Exercise three

Bust Lift

What it does
This very simple standing exercise will tone and lift the bust.

How to do it
Stand with your feet hip-width apart. Take a football (if you don't have one, scrunch a towel up into a ball shape), place your hands on either side of it and squeeze, holding the ball several inches away from your body at chest height. Maintaining the squeeze, extend the arms out fully then raise them a few inches. Hold, then lower and draw the arms back in, always applying pressure to the ball. Repeat for one minute.

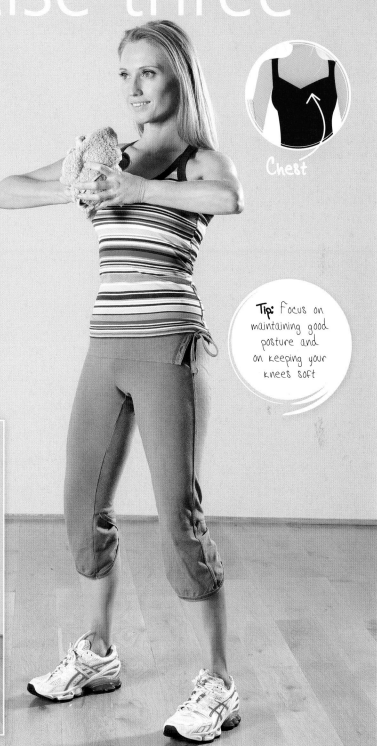

Chest

Tip: Focus on maintaining good posture and on keeping your knees soft

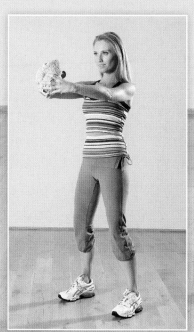

Exercise four

Luscious Legs

What it does
This exercise works the muscles of both your inner and outer legs. It's also a great way of increasing your hip flexibility, and the added bonus is that you use your abdominal muscles for control and balance.

How to do it
Lie face up on your towel or mat. Extend your legs straight up with your feet flexed and rest your arms out to the sides with your palms face down. Engage your abdominal muscles and simultaneously lower your legs slowly, one to each side. Hold, and then slowly draw them both back to the centre. Repeat for one minute.

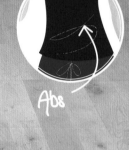

Thighs

Abs

Tip: Focus on keeping your stomach muscles pulled in tight throughout the exercise

Exercise five

Curvy Curves

What it does

This is one of my personal favourites as it targets all your abdominal muscles at once. Another great thing is that when you get fitter you can up the intensity by simply bringing your legs a little closer to the ground. It feels challenging but it's worth it for the results.

How to do it

Lie face up, knees raised so that they are above your hips, your fingertips behind your ears and your elbows bent. Raise your head, extend your right leg at 45° to the floor and raise the right side of your chest to meet your left knee. Switch legs and repeat. Continue alternating for one minute.

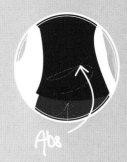

Abs

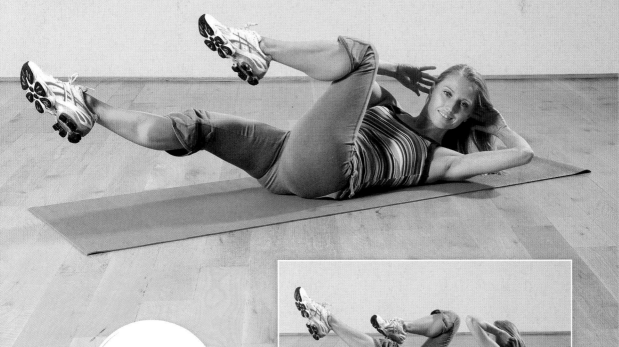

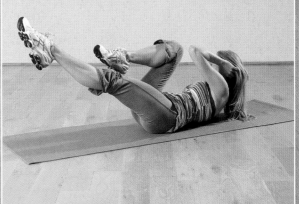

Tip: Keep your abs pulled in tight as you do this one to protect your back

MEAL PLAN
tuck in...

Monday	Tuesday

Breakfast
Omelette made with 2 egg whites and chopped peppers and tomatoes

Mid-morning snack
Handful of nuts and raisins

Lunch
Jacket potato with baked beans

Mid-afternoon snack
Carrot and celery sticks with butter bean pâté (simply mash up the butter beans to make the pâté)

Dinner
Grilled strips of chicken breast on ratatouille

Breakfast
Porridge with berries

Mid-morning snack
2 Ryvitas with cottage cheese and slices of ham

Lunch
Can of vegetable soup

Mid-afternoon snack
Metabolic calorie-burning smoothie (see p89)

Dinner
Homemade lentil curry served on brown rice

Eat small and regular

It's better to have five or six small meals a day than three large ones. This is because it helps to regulate your blood sugar levels, meaning your body is less likely to store fat

Wednesday

Breakfast
2 poached eggs with grilled mushrooms

Mid-morning snack
Banana and handful of berries

Lunch
Couscous with grated courgette, carrots and cucumber

Mid-afternoon snack
Sugar-free protein bar

Dinner
Vegetable stir-fry with lots of leafy green vegetables

Thursday

Breakfast
Wholegrain cereal with chopped banana

Mid-morning snack
2 oatcakes

Lunch
Sliced hard-boiled egg with tomatoes, onions, olives, avocado on a rocket salad

Mid-afternoon snack
Handful of homemade popcorn

Dinner
Grilled cod with toasted breadcrumbs served with spinach and small amount of mashed potato

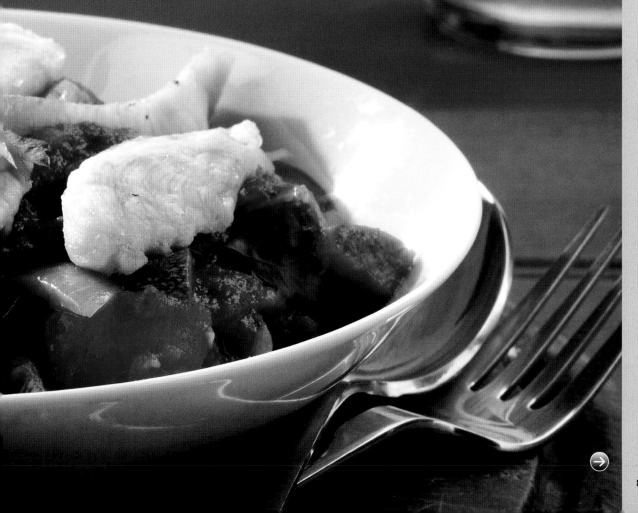

continued...

| **Friday** | **Saturday** | **Sunday** |

Breakfast
Metabolic calorie-burning smoothie (see p89)

Mid-morning snack
Carrot, pepper and cucumber sticks with low-fat cottage cheese

Lunch
Bean salad: kidney beans, haricot beans, chickpeas with chopped red onion in a little olive oil

Mid-afternoon snack
Handful of nuts and raisins

Dinner
Grilled lean pork chop served with mashed sweet potato and peas

Breakfast
2 scrambled eggs with grilled tomatoes and slice of wholemeal toast

Mid-morning snack
2 oatcakes topped with avocado

Lunch
Turkey slices with salad in a toasted wholemeal pitta

Mid-afternoon snack
Kiwi fruit with 150g pot of low-fat yoghurt

Dinner
Grilled salmon fillet topped with pesto served with 3 new potatoes and sweetcorn

Breakfast
Buckwheat pancakes served with low-fat fromage frais and berries

Mid-morning snack
Rice cake with peanut butter

Lunch
Tuna Niçoise salad

Mid-afternoon snack
Toasted crumpet with a drizzle of honey

Dinner
Lean beef mince topped with sweet potato mash, served with peas

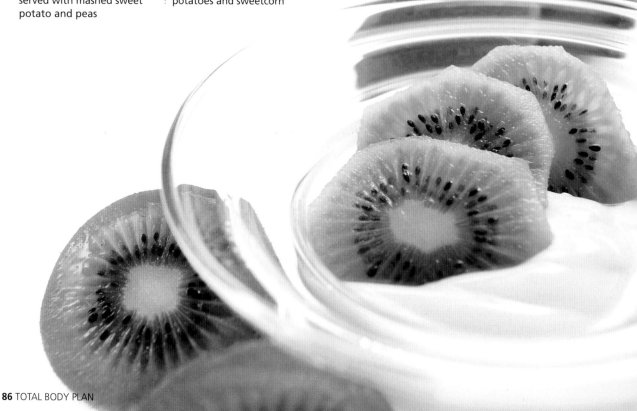

Shopping list

Wholemeal pittas, bread
Brown rice
Couscous
Lentils
Buckwheat flour
Ryvitas
Rice cakes
Crumpets
Oatcakes
Cereal, porridge oats
Popcorn
Nuts and raisins
Wheatgerm
Low-fat milk, yoghurts, fromage frais, cottage cheese
Tins of tuna, vegetable soup, tomatoes, butter beans, haricot beans, kidney beans, chickpeas, baked beans
Fruit/veg: aubergine, avocados, bananas, carrots, celery, courgettes, cucumber, fresh herbs, frozen berries, garlic, jacket potatoes, kiwi fruit, mushrooms, new potatoes, olives, onions, peas, peppers, red onion, salad leaves, spinach, strawberries, sweetcorn, sweet potatoes, tomatoes
Ham slices (cooked)
Turkey slices (cooked)
Salmon fillets
Cod steak
Chicken breasts
Lean steak mince
Lean pork chop
Eggs
Soy sauce, olive oil, curry powder, pesto
Honey, peanut butter
Sugar-free protein bar

Food facts
Jump-start your metabolism

From as early as a person's mid-twenties the metabolism – literally, the sum total of chemical processes that take place in the body – begins gradually to slow down. It's no surprise, then, that many women come to me and say, 'I'm putting on weight but I'm eating less.' The reason is that, the slower your metabolism becomes, the easier it is to gain weight because your body is now burning fewer calories.

But fear not. We can change all that by naturally increasing your metabolism on a daily basis. We do this in several ways. The first is by eating breakfast. For the past eight hours while you've been sleeping your body has gone into starvation mode: your metabolism has slowed down to conserve energy, otherwise known as calories. Having that healthy breakfast will rev it back up.

Eat smaller meals more frequently. Don't skip your mid-morning or mid-afternoon snacks as these will keep your blood sugar stable and provide a steady source of energy to fuel your metabolism.

Doing your circuits will ensure that your muscles are toned. And the more toned your muscles are the more calories they burn. Regular exercise not only burns calories during your workout, but also encourages your body to keep burning extra calories for up to two hours after you stop exercising.

Ensure your diet includes plenty of vitamin B5 – found in mushrooms, avocados, tomatoes, cabbage, eggs, whole wheat, peas and lentils – because this boosts your metabolic rate.

Stick to the above and you'll turn back your metabolic body clock to a time when you naturally burned more calories daily.

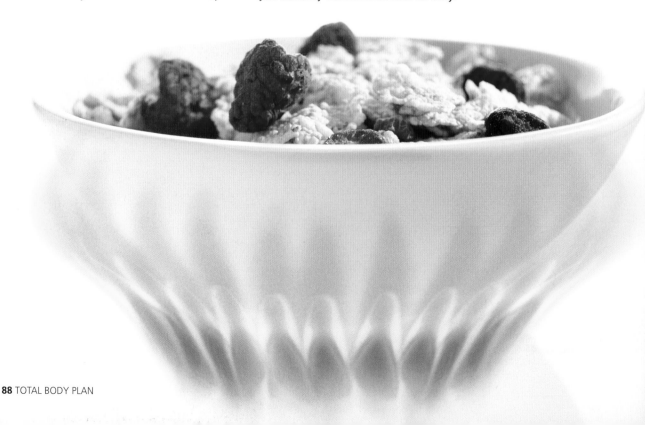

Blend it

Metabolic calorie-burning smoothie

This easy-to-make smoothie is packed full of fruit and vitamin B5, which will get your metabolism firing. It has the added benefit that the blend of nutrients will give you healthy skin and hair

Ingredients

* Handful of strawberries
* Avocado
* Stick of celery
* Glass of low-fat milk
* 1 tsp of wheatgerm

Chuck it all in a blender, whiz it and drink it

Soothing body wrap

Turn your home into a spa by creating your own hydrating and moisturising soothing body wrap. This will give tired skin a lift, leaving it feeling silky smooth. You'll be fresh and glowing all over – and all in the comfort of your own home.

What you need

* A blender
* Cucumber
* Bunch of mint leaves
* Aloe vera gel
* Lavender and chamomile essential oils
* Clingfilm

What to do

* Put a quarter of a cucumber and a handful of chopped mint leaves into the blender. Add two tablespoons of aloe vera gel and five drops each of the lavender and chamomile essential oils, then whiz to form a paste.

* Refrigerate for 30 minutes then spread on thighs, bottom, tummy and chest. Cover with clingfilm to help the hydrating mask soak in, relax for 15 minutes, then rinse off.

* To maintain your healthy glow, apply twice a week.

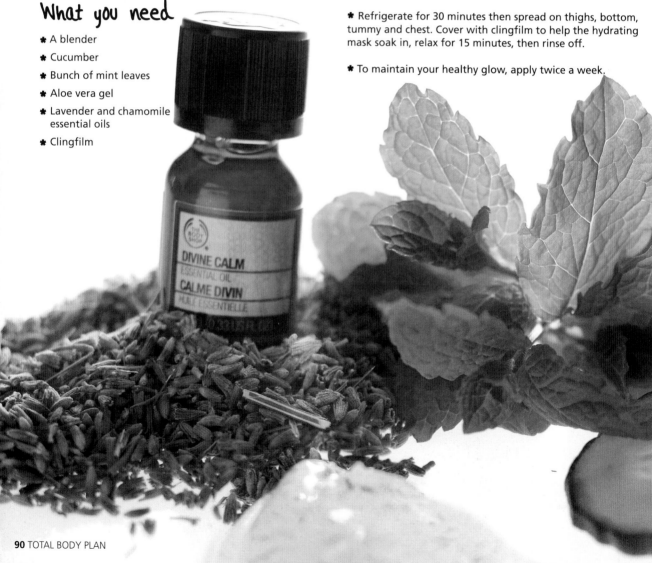

Q&A

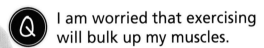

YOUR QUESTIONS ANSWERED

Q I am a classic pear shape. How can I rid myself of the stubborn fat around my hips and thighs?

A: Unfortunately, you can't 'spot reduce' or target an area with a specific exercise to reduce body fat. You can only get rid of fat from everywhere by watching your diet, burning off calories through exercise and increasing your metabolism by training your muscles – all of which this plan will do. Women tend to store fat around their hips and thighs (with men, it's the belly) so if you lose fat, these will be the areas where it shows most.

Q I am worried that exercising will bulk up my muscles.

A: Doing this plan will increase your muscle tissue, but this takes up less space than flabby muscles or the same amount of fat. All the exercises designed in this programme will tone, define and lengthen your muscles. You will not bulk up.

Q Is there a best time of the day to train?

A: The answer to this is down to the individual. If you are an early bird and are good in the mornings, then this is a great time to do your exercise. Some people feel more alert and motivated later in the day – I always prefer to train in the afternoon. It's a personal choice. Choose the time of day that suits you best and make that your regular workout time. It'll become a habit you stick to.

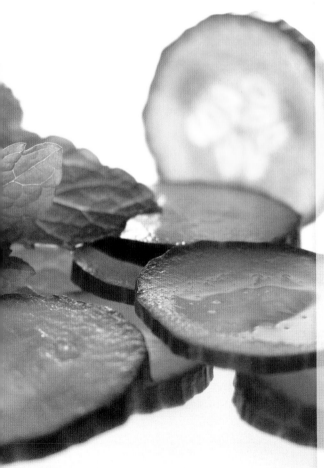

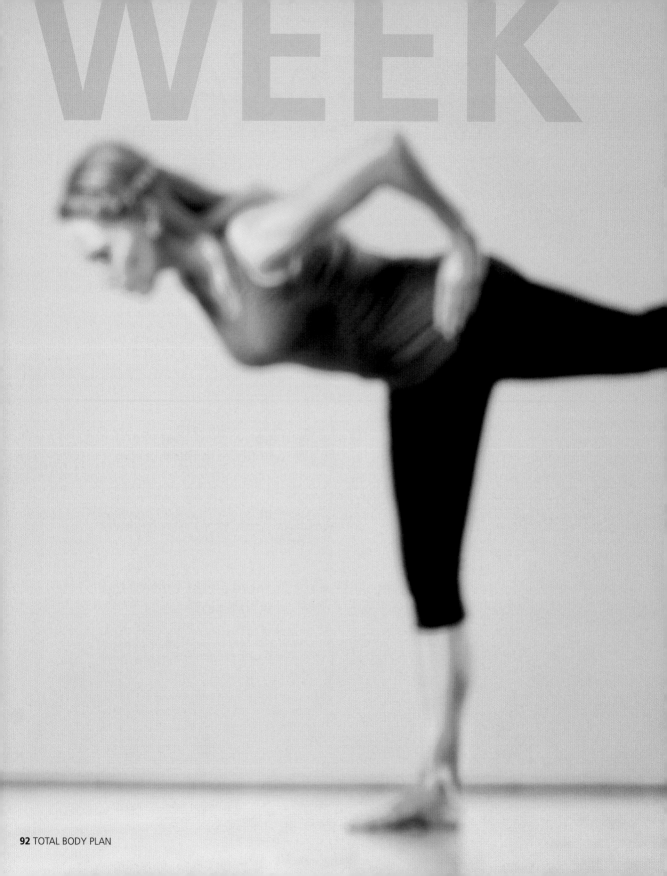

FIVE

'Spend 15 minutes to spend the rest of the day feeling fantastic'

WEEK FIVE

the plan...

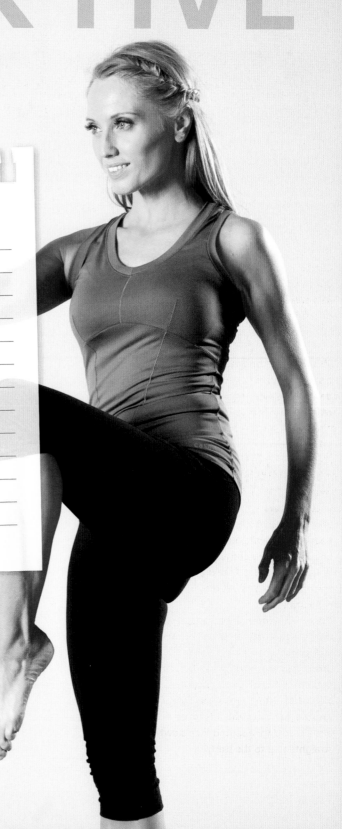

Monday 15-minute fast firm-up see opposite

Tuesday 1 x home circuit see p96

Wednesday 15-minute fast firm-up

Thursday 1 x home circuit

Friday 15-minute fast firm-up

Saturday 2 x home circuits

Sunday Rest

TOP TIP
When doing your squats, keep movements slow. This will tone deep into your glutes. Make sure too that your knees don't shoot out over your toes

Aerobic
15-minute fast firm-up

Week Five is going to firm you up all over and tighten up those troublesome areas: the thighs, hips, bottom and abs. Combining six moves that can be done indoors or al fresco, it will also naturally increase the amount of calories your body burns.

How to do it
This workout consists of four exercises, plus marching and jogging on the spot. With any exercise that requires your feet to leave the floor, always be sure to land softly.

* **Calf raises**
Standing with good posture, raise yourself up on to your toes, then lower.

* **Crossovers**
Standing with good posture, keeping your back straight, lift your left knee and bring your right elbow to touch it. Return to the start then switch to the right knee and left elbow.

* **Shuttle runs**
Place two markers approximately 20 metres apart and run between them.

* **Squats**
Stand with your feet hip-width apart, feeling the weight through your heels. Breathe in, then exhale and bend as if you are about to sit on a chair. Hold for a second then slowly straighten up to the start.

Time (mins)	Exercise	Perceived rate of exertion
0-1	March on the spot	3-4
1-3	Jog on the spot, knees high	6
3-4	Calf raises	5
4-5	Crossovers	5
5-6	Shuttle runs	6
6-7	Squats	5
7-8	Jog on the spot, knees high	6
8-9	Calf raises	6
9-10	Crossovers	5
10-11	Shuttle runs	6
11-12	Squats	5
12-14	Jog on the spot, knees high	6
14-15	March on the spot to cool down	5

Home circuits
Just ten minutes

Warm up for two to three minutes (see p18), then perform the five exercises in order. Do each for one minute before moving straight on to the next with no rest in between. Once you've finished spend two minutes doing some stretching (see p19)

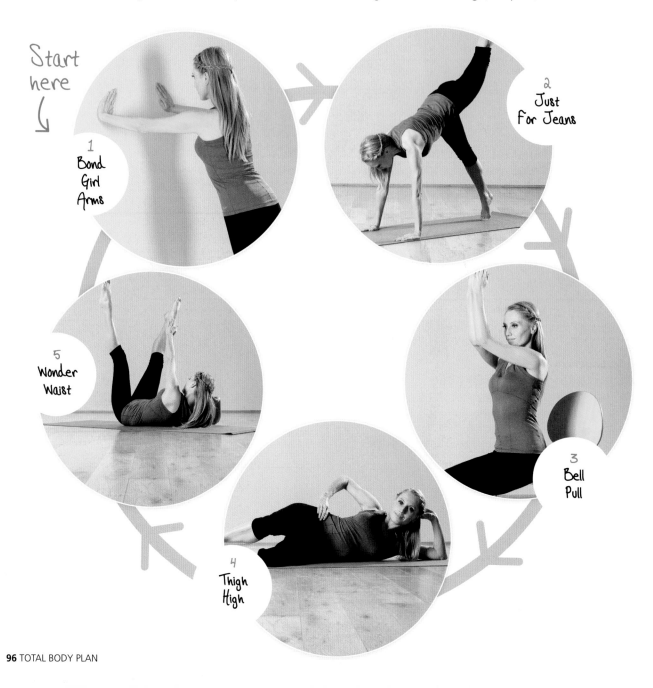

Start here ↓

1
Bond Girl Arms

2
Just For Jeans

3
Bell Pull

4
Thigh High

5
Wonder Waist

Exercise one

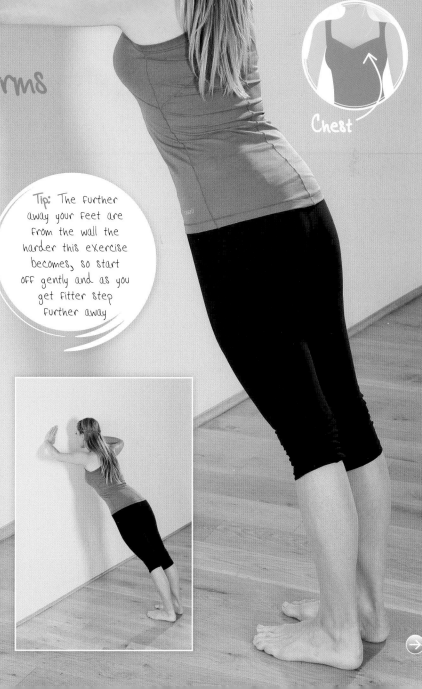

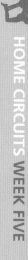

Arms

Chest

Bond Girl Arms

What it does
This standing exercise gives your upper arms a fantastic workout, toning and sculpting the triceps.

How to do it
Place your hands on the wall a little lower than shoulder level, with your thumb and first finger turned in slightly towards each other. Your elbows should be wider than shoulder-width, and your feet should be at least six inches away from the wall so that your weight is through your hands. Slowly bend your elbows to lower yourself towards the wall, then push yourself back up to a straight-arm position. Continue for one minute.

Tip: The further away your feet are from the wall the harder this exercise becomes, so start off gently and as you get fitter step further away

Exercise two

Just For Jeans

What it does

The clever thing with this yoga-inspired move is that, while you're toning one leg, you're stretching through the back of the other. You'll feel long and lean afterwards.

How to do it

On all fours on the floor, push your bottom up so you form an upside-down V shape. Keep your abdominals pulled in tight to protect your back, make sure your feet are hip-width apart and your hands are under your shoulders. Slowly raise one leg behind you, keeping it straight and pointing the toes. Squeeze your bottom muscles tight, hold for a second, then slowly lower the leg. Switch legs and continue for one minute.

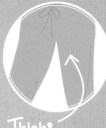

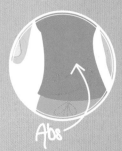

Thighs

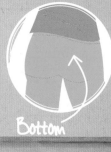

Abs

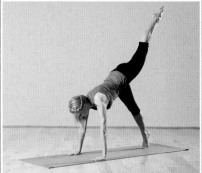

Bottom

Tip: Keep this exercise slow and controlled

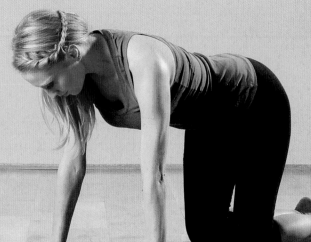

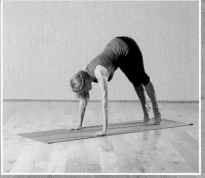

Exercise three

Bell Pull

What it does
This sitting exercise works your bust and the backs of your upper arms at the same time.

How to do it
Sit on a chair with good posture, feet hip-width apart. Lift your arms to shoulder level and bend your elbows to a 90° angle. Press elbows, forearms and hands together and lift your hands towards the ceiling, keeping your forearms pressed together. Slowly lower the elbows back to start. Do this for one minute.

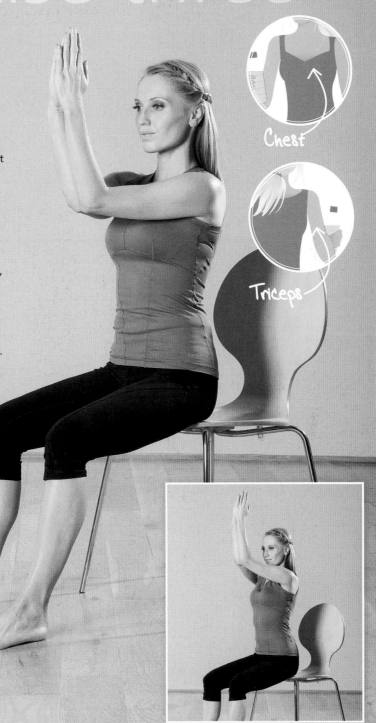

Chest

Triceps

Tip: Ensure you keep your elbows at chest height. If you drop too low it will reduce the effectiveness of the exercise

Exercise four

Thigh High

What it does
Tones deep into your inner thigh muscles, which will sculpt your legs, giving you great definition and allowing you to slip into your shorts with confidence.

How to do it
Lying on your side with your body in a straight line, bring your thighs up slightly in front of you, with your knees bent. Support your head with your bottom arm and have your top arm bent with hand on hip for balance. Keeping your heels together, slowly turn your top leg out slightly so you're rotating your hip. Hold for a couple of seconds, then turn it in halfway, before turning it out again. Do this for 30 seconds on each side.

Thighs

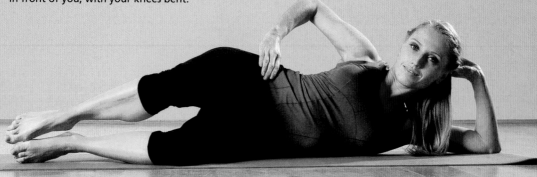

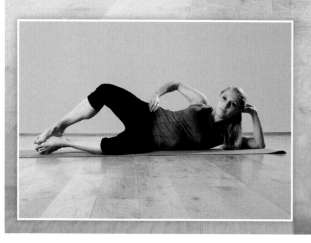

Tip: To work the leg harder imagine you are having to lift the leg up against resistance. It's amazing how this little trick of the mind can increase the intensity of this exercise

Exercise five

Wonder Waist

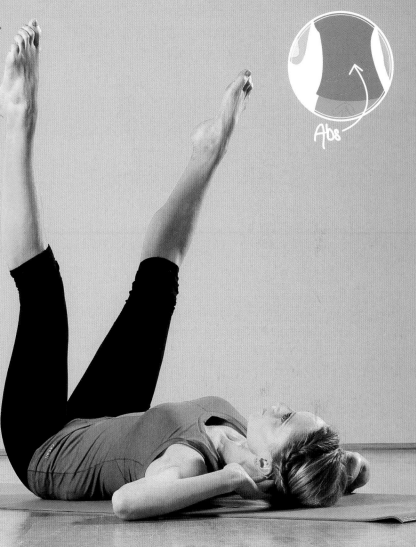

Abs

What it does
Encourages you to work all your abdominal muscles in one move. By aiming to touch your leg you'll ensure you are working through a good range of movement, which will give you a wonder waist.

How to do it
Lie on your back on your mat with your legs extended but parted slightly so that your toes are shoulder-width apart. Place your fingertips by your ears and lift both shoulders off the floor, before reaching with your right hand towards your left foot, keeping your abs pulled in tight. Slowly lower your hand and repeat with the left hand aiming to reach the right foot. Continue for one minute.

Tip: Keep your legs in line with your hips

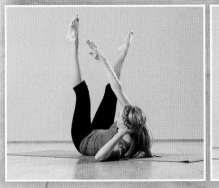

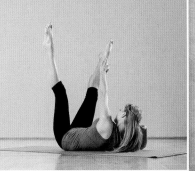

101

tuck in...

Monday	Tuesday

Breakfast
Muesli with dried apricots

Mid-morning snack
Sliced avocado and small slice of mozzarella

Lunch
Tuna salad sandwich on wholemeal bread

Mid-afternoon snack
Carrot and celery sticks with butter bean pâté (simply mash up the butter beans to make the pâté)

Dinner
King prawn stir-fry with vegetables and rice noodles

Breakfast
Wholemeal muffin with poached egg

Mid-morning snack
Banana with handful of raisins

Lunch
Jacket potato with tuna or cottage cheese and side salad

Mid-afternoon snack
Apple

Dinner
Steamed salmon with asparagus and new potato

Don't shop on an empty stomach

Have a snack before you visit the supermarket. You'll be less tempted to put fattening treats in your trolley

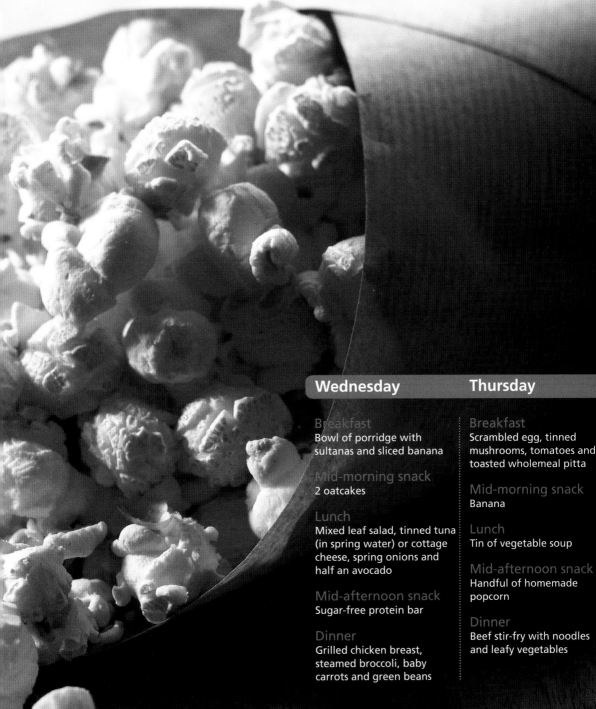

Wednesday

Breakfast
Bowl of porridge with
sultanas and sliced banana

Mid-morning snack
2 oatcakes

Lunch
Mixed leaf salad, tinned tuna
(in spring water) or cottage
cheese, spring onions and
half an avocado

Mid-afternoon snack
Sugar-free protein bar

Dinner
Grilled chicken breast,
steamed broccoli, baby
carrots and green beans

Thursday

Breakfast
Scrambled egg, tinned
mushrooms, tomatoes and
toasted wholemeal pitta

Mid-morning snack
Banana

Lunch
Tin of vegetable soup

Mid-afternoon snack
Handful of homemade
popcorn

Dinner
Beef stir-fry with noodles
and leafy vegetables

Friday

Breakfast
Boiled egg with
wholemeal toast

Mid-morning snack
Ryvita with butter bean pâté

Lunch
Tuna and red kidney bean
salad with red onion

Mid-afternoon snack
Handful of nuts and raisins

Dinner
Spaghetti Bolognese made
with lean mince and
wholemeal spaghetti

Saturday

Breakfast
Hydrating smoothie
(see p107)

Mid-morning snack
Handful popcorn

Lunch
Small jacket potato with
low-fat cottage cheese and
pineapple chunks

Mid-afternoon snack
Kiwi fruit with 150g pot
of low-fat yoghurt

Dinner
Grilled beef steak with
grilled tomatoes, served
with salad

Sunday

Breakfast
Mixed berries with 150g
pot of low-fat yoghurt and
porridge oats

Mid-morning snack
Slice of wholemeal toast
with drizzle of honey

Lunch
Grilled chicken breast with
couscous and mixed peppers

Mid-afternoon snack
Toasted crumpet with
a drizzle of honey

Dinner
Wholemeal pasta with
steamed broccoli, tinned
pink salmon and low-fat soft
cream cheese with herbs

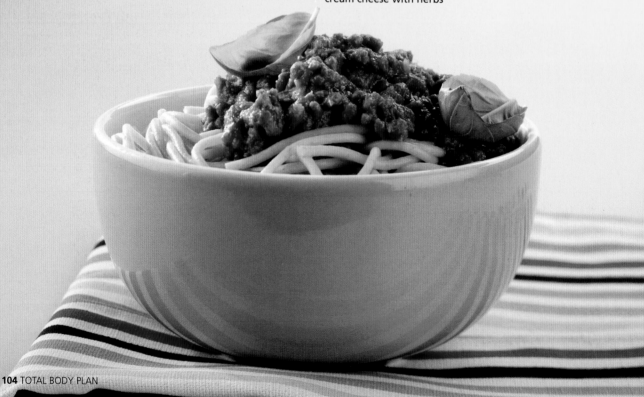

Shopping list

Wholemeal spaghetti, penne pasta, pittas, bread, muffins

Crumpets, for toasting

Rice noodles

Couscous

Oatcakes

Tins of tuna, pink salmon, vegetable soup, tomatoes, butter beans, kidney beans, mushrooms, pineapple chunks

Ryvitas

Porridge oats

Muesli

Nuts, raisins, sultanas

Fruit/veg: apples, asparagus, avocados, baby carrots, bananas, broccoli, cucumber, frozen berries, jacket potatoes, kiwi fruit, new potatoes, peppers, red onion, salad leaves, spring onions, sweet potatoes, tomatoes, watermelon

Salmon fillets

King prawns

Chicken breasts

Lean steak mince

Lean beef steaks

Low-fat yoghurts, cottage cheese, mozzarella, soft cream cheese with herbs

Eggs

Sugar-free protein bar

The wonders of water

We've heard it a million times, that we have to drink our eight glasses of water a day. Yet it can seem like a chore. But there are ways of ensuring that by the end of play each day your water levels are fully topped up.

The benefits to being fully hydrated are endless. Drinking your eight a day will give you more energy, plump up your skin, lubricate your joints, help to flatten your tummy (believe it or not, drinking water can help beat water retention) and it will improve your body's ability to burn calories. This simple and totally accessible drink really is a wonder tonic.

The key to getting all you need of it is a little bit of discipline and routine. Just get into the following habits…

Always have a glass with your breakfast. You could have this hot with a slice of lemon, which is a great way to wake you up and works well as a detox. So, seven to go.

Have two glasses with your mid-morning snack. This will rev up your energy levels and keep you alert. At lunch have a large glass – so you really are having two in one – with a very small amount of sugar-free juice in it.

Only three glasses to go now – this is looking like an achievable healthy new habit. With your mid-afternoon snack have two glasses. Again, this will keep you energised throughout the afternoon. Your last glass can be enjoyed with your evening meal – add some ice for a little variety.

As part of your Total Body Plan, I also recommend that at the end of both your aerobic workouts and your circuits you drink plenty of water to keep your body cool and hydrated. Here's to your new habit of eight glasses a day.

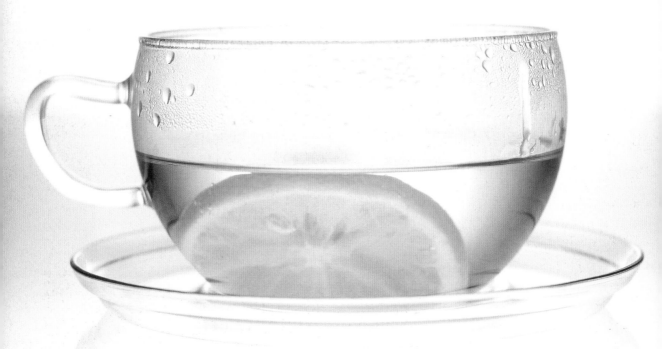

Blend it
Hydrating smoothie

A mouthwatering smoothie – cucumber and watermelon make this hydrating and incredibly refreshing. It also helps maintain fluid balance in the body, with the bonus that it will keep your skin plumped up and hydrated

Ingredients

- Half a watermelon
- Half an unpeeled cucumber
- 5 crushed ice cubes
- 2 tbsp of soya milk
- 1 tsp of honey

Chuck it all in a blender, whiz it and drink it

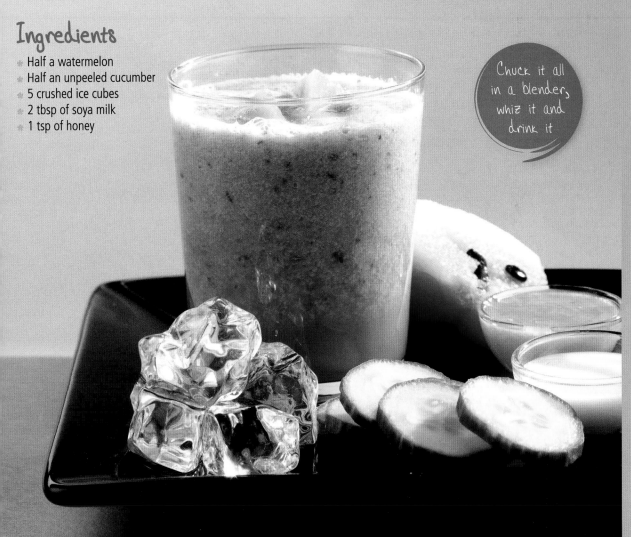

Look great

Olive oil hair mask

Treat yourself to this easy-to-make hair mask that will leave your hair feeling super-soft and shiny. If you eat lots of fruit and vegetables and do your exercises, you will notice that your hair becomes healthier and looks better – and this hair mask will give it an extra boost.

What you need

* 5 tbps of olive oil
* 2 eggs

How to do it

Simply mix the olive oil and eggs together in a bowl. Wash your hair with your normal shampoo, rinse, then apply the mask all over your damp hair. Massage thoroughly, then cover it with a towel or a shower hat. Your body heat will help the mask to penetrate. Leave for a minimum of 30 minutes, then shampoo out, rinsing well.

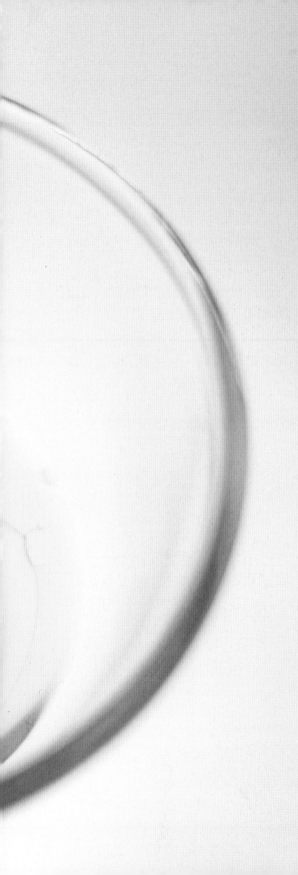

Q&A

YOUR QUESTIONS ANSWERED

Q Sometimes I don't stretch after a workout. Is this OK?

A: It is important always to stretch after your workout. The purpose of stretching is to keep your muscles healthy – it will prevent soreness and injuries. To get the full benefit of your workout, always finish off by stretching.

Q With toning exercises, is it better to do more reps fast, say doing hundreds of sit-ups, or am I better doing fewer and slowly?

A: Quality is far better for your muscles that quantity. Performing toning exercises quickly develops a momentum, so the muscles don't get to train as hard, which means the exercise is less effective. I always encourage my clients to do all their circuit toning moves slowly – it means the muscles are working longer and harder. Twenty slow reps is far better than 100 fast.

Q How can I stick to the full six-week programme without giving up?

A: The programme is designed to be easy to fit into your lifestyle, so that it's time-friendly and achievable. You'll feel great every time you exercise, and the combined results of your body looking good and you feeling good will mean that you now enjoy exercising. It'll no longer be a chore.

WEEK

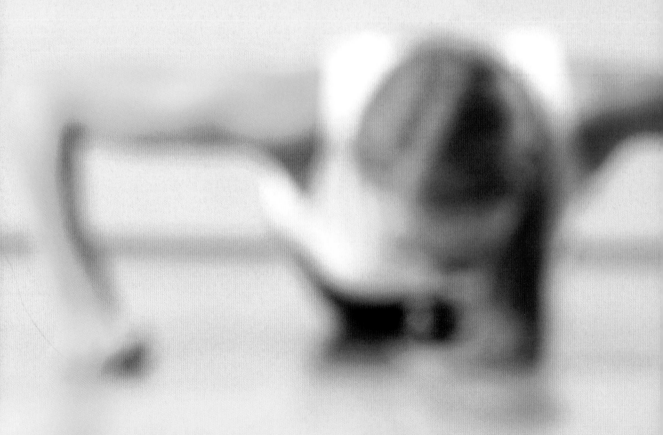

SIX

'There are no side effects to fitness, only the benefits of looking and feeling great'

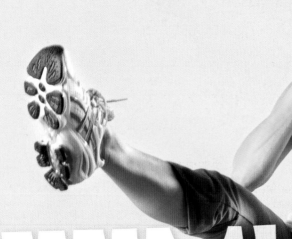

WEEK SIX
the plan...

Monday 15-minute kick box see opposite

Tuesday 1 x home circuit see p114

Wednesday 15-minute kick box

Thursday 1 x home circuit

Friday 15-minute kick box

Saturday 2 x home circuits

Sunday Rest

TOP TIP
Don't over-extend your kicks or lock your joints. Always keep your tummy muscles pulled in when you are doing your kicks and jabs as this will give you an incredible abdominal workout

Aerobic
15-minute kick box

You've made it to Week Six. Well done. Now this fun-filled, high-energy workout is going to get your heart pumping and give you a full-body workout.

How to do it

When marching and jogging on the spot always make sure you land softly and keep the knees slightly bent. For the kick-boxing moves, do like this:

* Front kick

Stand with feet shoulder-width apart. Bend your knees slightly, and pull your right knee up toward your chest. Point your knee in the direction of an imaginary target, then kick out with the ball of your foot. Repeat with your other leg

* Skipping

This can be done with a skipping rope, or simply mimic the movement without the rope.

* Jab

Stand with your feet hip-width apart, knees soft and hips facing forwards. Punch your arms out in front of you at chest height, alternating the arms and keeping your abs pulled in tight to keep your lower body solid.

Time (mins)	Exercise	Perceived rate of exertion
0-2	March on the spot	3-4
2-3	Front kick on right leg	5
3-4	Front kick on left leg	5
4-5	Skipping	6
5-6	Jab	6
6-7	Jog on the spot	6
7-8	Front kick on the right leg	5
8-9	Front kick on the left leg	5
9-10	Jab	6
10-11	Jog on the spot	6
11-12	Front kick on the right leg	5
12-14	Front kick on the left leg	5
14-15	March on the spot to cool down	4

Home circuits
Just ten minutes

Warm up for two to three minutes (see p18), then perform the five exercises in order. Do each for one minute before moving straight on to the next with no rest in between. Once you've finished spend two minutes doing some stretching (see p19)

Start here ↓

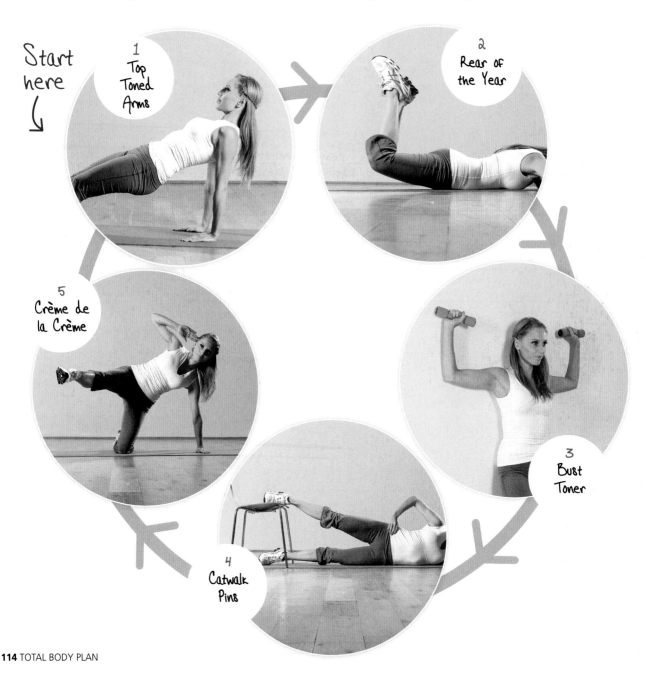

1 Top Toned Arms

2 Rear of the Year

3 Bust Toner

4 Catwalk Pins

5 Crème de la Crème

Exercise one

Top toned arms

What it does
This is a challenging exercise but fantastic for sculpting your upper arms as it really works your triceps.

How to do it
Sit on the floor with legs straight and together. Place your hands, fingertips forwards, just behind your hips and point your toes. Pull in your abs, then straighten your arms (your hands should be under your shoulders) and lift your hips off the floor until your body is in a line from shoulders to toes. Hold for several seconds then slowly lower your hips. Rest for a couple of seconds, then repeat. Do this for one minute.

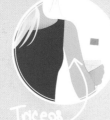

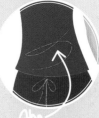
Triceps

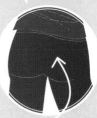
Abs

Bottom

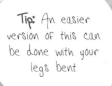
Tip: An easier version of this can be done with your legs bent

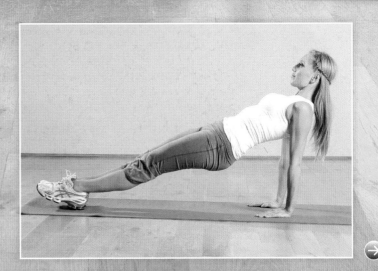

Exercise two

Rear of the Year

What it does

This fabulous floor exercise gives you a bottom lift that you will be proud to show off. You'll feel this one working straightaway.

How to do it

Lying face down on the floor, bend your knees and place your heels together. Slowly separate your knees until they are several inches apart, while keeping your heels together. Keep your upper body firmly on the floor. With your head resting on your hands, aim to lift your thighs several inches off the floor by squeezing tightly into your buttocks. Hold this for a couple of seconds then slowly lower. Repeat for one minute.

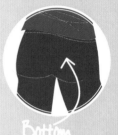

Bottom

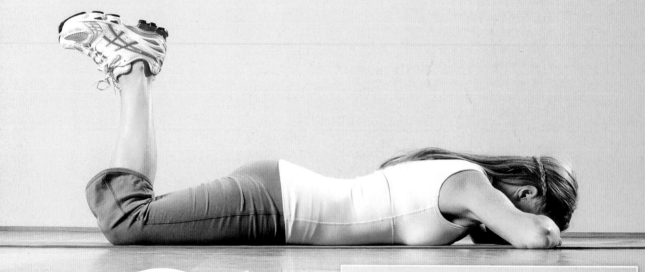

Tip: If you want to train a little harder, see if you can hold the squeeze for five seconds

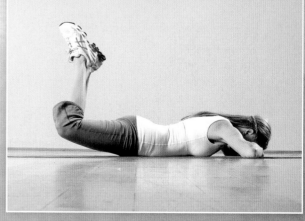

Exercise three

Bust Toner

What it does

Tones the pectoralis major – which support the bust – and works your triceps.

How to do it

Stand with your back pressed to the wall, feet 12 inches in front of you with knees slightly bent. Holding your hand weights, lift your elbows to shoulder height, forearms at right angles, all still in contact with the wall. Take a deep breath and, as you breathe out, bring both arms in so your forearms meet in the middle. Breathe in and return to the start. To get your abs working on this one, keep your belly button pulled tight to the spine. Be sure not to let the back arch. Do this for one minute.

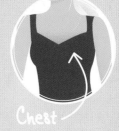

Chest

Tip: Make sure you keep your elbows in line with your shoulders

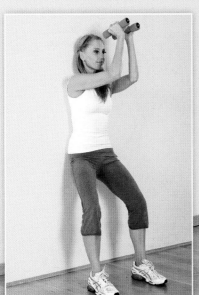

Exercise four

Catwalk Pins

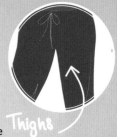

Thighs

What it does

This side-lying exercise will give tone and shape to your thighs, at the same time stretching the muscles. Before long, if you stick to it, you'll have lovely, long, lean legs. Using the chair encourages you to work through a bigger range of movement.

How to do it

Lie on your side and support your head with one hand. Lift your top leg and place your foot on the chair. Very slowly, lift the lower leg to touch the underside of the chair, hold for a few seconds, lower several inches, then lift straight back. Continue for 30 seconds then switch legs and repeat.

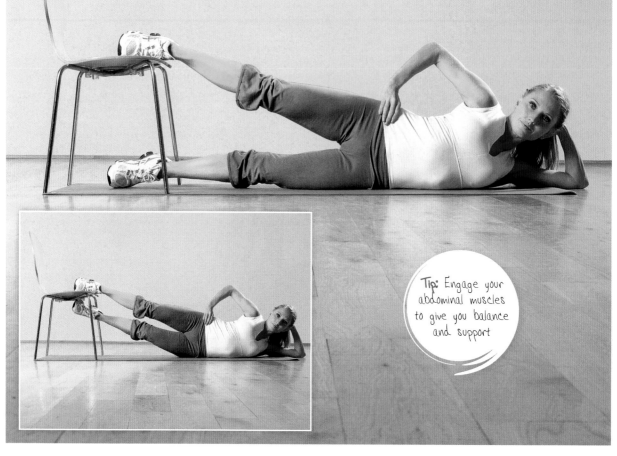

Tip: Engage your abdominal muscles to give you balance and support

Exercise five

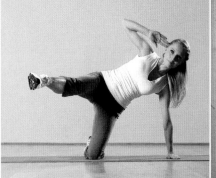

Tip: Aim to keep your upper body perfectly still as you perform this. Do this by engaging your abdominal muscles by pulling them in tight

Crème de la Crème

What it does

This is quite a challenging exercise, as it tests your balance while it tones deep into your abdominal muscles. It's worth it though – you'll see and feel it working immediately.

How to do it

Kneel on the floor on your mat, and lean all the way over to your left side, placing your left palm on the floor. Keeping your weight balanced, slowly extend your right leg and point your toes. Place your right hand behind your head, pointing your elbow towards the ceiling. Slowly lift your leg to hip height, at the same time pull in your abdominal muscles, then very slowly swing your right leg out in front of you, maintaining the same height. Hold, then bring the leg back so you are in a straight line. Aim to repeat this for 30 seconds, then rest and change sides.

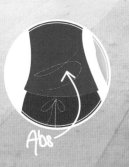

Abs

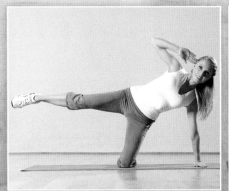

tuck in...

Monday

Breakfast
Porridge with
sprinkled cinnamon

Mid-morning snack
Ryvita with cottage cheese
and apple

Lunch
Sardines on wholemeal toast

Mid-afternoon snack
Banana and seeds

Dinner
Chicken casserole with beans,
lentils, chickpeas, celery,
onions and garlic, served
with brown rice

Tuesday

Breakfast
Rainbow smoothie
(see p125)

Mid-morning snack
Sliced courgette, carrot, and
celery with cottage cheese

Lunch
Can of vegetable soup with
added brown rice

Mid-afternoon snack
Toasted crumpet with
drizzle of honey

Dinner
Grilled lean beef steak with
roasted vegetables

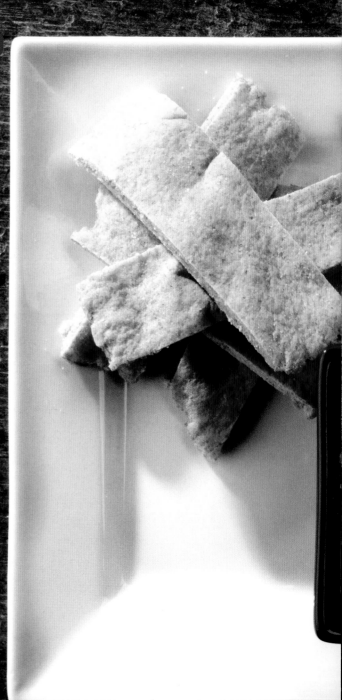

Drink before you snack

If you're feeling hungry, take a drink first. Thirst can sometimes be mistaken for hunger, and a glass of water can remove those temptations to raid the biscuit barrel

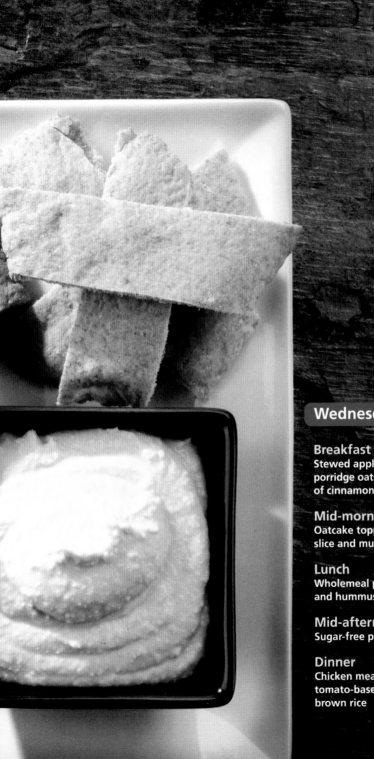

Wednesday

Breakfast
Stewed apple with porridge oats and sprinkling of cinnamon

Mid-morning snack
Oatcake topped with ham slice and mustard

Lunch
Wholemeal pitta with salad and hummus

Mid-afternoon snack
Sugar-free protein bar

Dinner
Chicken meatballs with tomato-based sauce on brown rice

Thursday

Breakfast
Grilled mushrooms on wholemeal toast

Mid-morning snack
Banana

Lunch
Avocado and sweetcorn brown rice salad

Mid-afternoon snack
Small slice of cheese with apple

Dinner
Wholemeal penne pasta with pesto and salad

MEAL PLAN

continued...

Friday	Saturday	Sunday

Breakfast
150g pot of low-fat yoghurt, berries and oats

Mid-morning snack
Hard-boiled egg with carrot batons

Lunch
Tuna and red kidney bean salad with red onion

Mid-afternoon snack
Handful of nuts and raisins

Dinner
Grilled salmon topped with pesto mixed with breadcrumbs and parmesan, served with salad leaves and sliced avocado

Breakfast
Crushed raspberries, on low fat crème fraîche on 2 slices of wholemeal toast

Mid-morning snack
Oatcakes with hummus

Lunch
Tbsp each of kidney beans, chickpeas and cannellini beans, red onion, tomatoes, olive oil, lemon , black pepper, wholemeal roll

Mid-afternoon snack
150g pot of low-fat yoghurt

Dinner
Salmon fish pie topped with sweet potato

Breakfast
Rainbow smoothie (see p125)

Mid-morning snack
Sliced peppers with low-fat cottage cheese

Lunch
Plum tomatoes on a slice of wholemeal toast with a little grated cheese

Mid-afternoon snack
Toasted crumpet with a drizzle of honey

Dinner
Cod fillet with tomato sauce on a bed of brown basmati rice with grilled vegetables

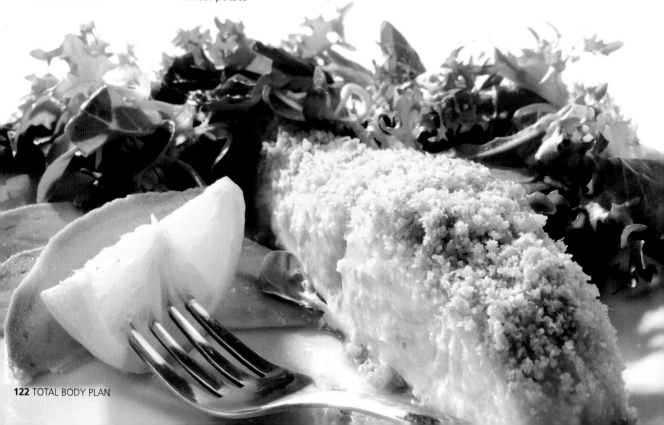

Shopping list

Wholemeal penne pasta, pittas, bread, rice
Crumpets, for toasting
Oatcakes
Ryvita
Porridge oats
Lentils
Nuts and raisins
Mixed seeds
Fruit/veg: apples, avocados, bananas, carrots, celery, courgettes, frozen berries, garlic, kiwi, mushrooms, onions, oranges, peppers, red onions, sweet potatoes, salad leaves, sweetcorn, tomatoes
Ham slices (cooked)
Salmon fillets
Cod fillet
Chicken breasts
Lean beef steak
Low-fat yoghurts, crème fraîche, cottage cheese, hummus, hard cheese, parmesan
Eggs
Tins of tuna, sardines, vegetable soup, tomatoes, butter beans, cannellini beans, kidney beans, chickpeas
Honey
Mustard
Pesto
Cinnamon
Sugar-free protein bar

Food facts
Eat a rainbow

Most of us know that it's important to eat at least five servings of fruits and vegetables every day. Yet we should also be aiming to have five different-coloured fruits and vegetables in our daily diet, the reason being that eating different-coloured fruit and veg provides us with the best all-round health benefits.

Each colour group contains different vitamins and nutrients, so having a rainbow of colours means you are guaranteed to get the range of essential vitamins and minerals – not only great for preventing disease but to give you great skin, hair, nails and heaps of energy.

Here are the colour groups and examples of the fruit and veg they contain…
Red: tomatoes, cherries, raspberries, red apples, strawberries, red peppers, rhubarb, red onions.
Yellow/orange: apricots, sweetcorn, carrots, mangoes, pumpkin, oranges, butternut squash, nectarines, sweet potato.
Blue: blueberries, aubergines, grapes, prunes, plums, pomegranates, purple cabbage.
Green: green beans, lettuce, spinach, broccoli, celery, green apples, courgettes, grapes, kiwi fruit.
White: cauliflower, turnips, parsnips, mushrooms, potatoes, onions, bananas.

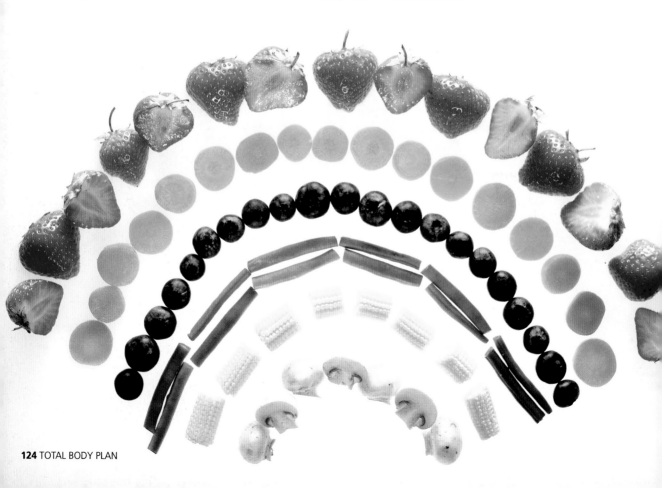

Blend it
Rainbow smoothie

This enticing, colourful smoothie contains five different-coloured fruits. Bursting with vitamins, minerals and powerful nutrients, it will brighten your day

Ingredients

* Banana, peeled
* Kiwi fruit, peeled
* Orange, peeled
* Handful of strawberries
* Handful of blueberries
* 150g pot of low-fat yoghurt

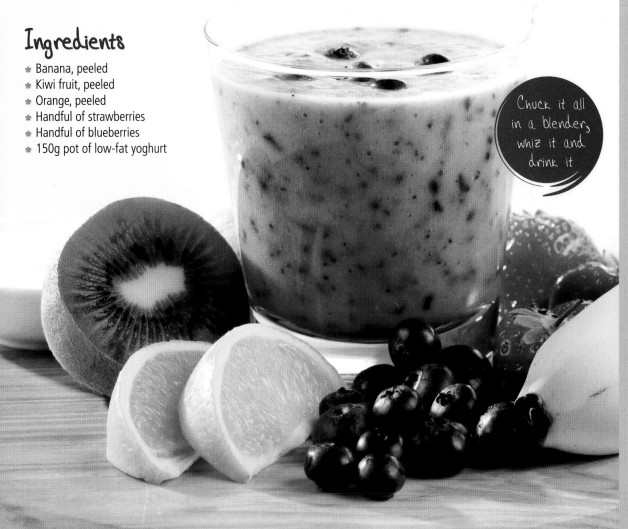

Chuck it all in a blender, whiz it and drink it

Look great
Treat yourself

Pampering yourself on a regular basis is a great way to boost your self-confidence. Think how much better you feel when you've had a nice manicure or pedicure – you instantly feel glamorous. It's not about spending a fortune on yourself, it's about recognising that treating yourself will increase that feel-good factor. A great way of doing this that won't cost a penny is a luxurious bath.

All you need is time at the end of the day to lock the bathroom door and completely switch off. Light a few candles around the bath, add a few drops of milk to the running water (they say that Cleopatra bathed in milk to preserve her legendary beauty) and a few drops of oil, then finish of by holding a teaspoon of honey under the tap. Now switch off the lights, submerge yourself in your five-star bath and unwind…

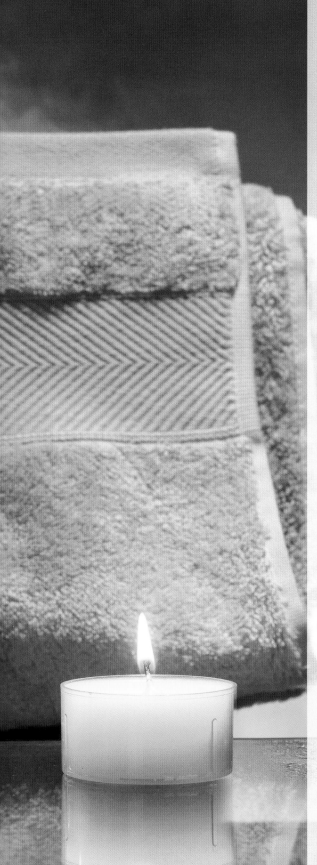

Q&A
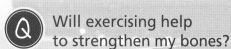

YOUR QUESTIONS ANSWERED

Q Will exercising help to strengthen my bones?

A: Your circuits involve toning exercises, which are also known as weight bearing exercises. These not only tone your muscles but also help to increase the density and strength of your bones.

Q Is exercising a good way of reducing stress?

A: One of the best ways of reducing stress is simply to exercise. Exercise will enhance your mood and it's a great way of motivating your mind.

Q I have a weakness for chocolate. Is it OK to sometimes have a little treat?

A: Yes, of course. We need to be realistic – the occasional treat is fine. It becomes a problem if, say, you do it every day. So I say to my clients, in any given week focus on being good 80% of the time, then 20% of the time you can have that odd little treat. If you find you can't resist that bar of chocolate, and your conscience bothers you, then compensate by doing an extra set of circuits.

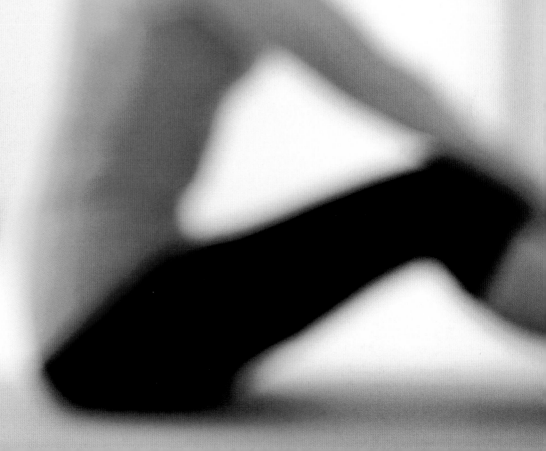

POSTNATAL
six-week plan

'Love the body you are in, and it will love you right back'

Postnatal
the plan...

Congratulations on your baby! That little bundle will take up most of your time from now on, but this plan is designed to fit around your busy life to get you back into great shape in just six weeks.

Straight after giving birth you don't want to place too much stress on your body, so the first two weeks of the plan use gentle exercises that will start to knit back your abdominal muscles and strengthen your pelvic floor while improving your body's natural alignment.

Weeks three and four add new exercises to help lift your bust and tone your abs and legs. Then, in the final two weeks, you'll progress on to exercises that firm up all the other parts of your body. At the end of six weeks, you'll be feeling fit, full of energy and looking great.

Power Pram Walks

As well as the home circuits, you'll do several Power Pram Walks each week. These will add a cardio element to your workout and get you and your baby out in the fresh air.

Remember to take water with you, and ensure the pram handles are at hip height to avoid leaning over. Walk tall with your tummy muscles pulled in.

Need inspiration? Get Lucy's audio coaching guide by downloading The LWR Postnatal Weight Loss Plan from iTunes and other online music stores

Power Pram Walks

Time (minutes)	Exercise	Rate of Perceived Exertion*
Week 1-2	**12-minute Power Pram Walk**	
0-1	Gentle	3
1-2	A little faster	5
2-3	Gentle	3
3-4	A little faster	5
4-6	Moderate pace, with 10 seconds on and off keeping your belly button pulled in tight	4
6-9	A little faster	5
9-11	Moderate pace	4
11-12	Gentle	3
Week 3-4	**Add these extra 4 minutes**	
12-14	Moderate pace, with 10 seconds on and off keeping your belly button pulled in tight	4
14-16	Gentle	3
Week 5-6	**Add these extra 8 minutes**	
16-19	A little faster	5
19-21	Moderate to fast pace, with 10 seconds on and off keeping your belly button pulled in tight	5
21-23	A little faster	5
23-24	Gentle	3

*Where 1 is barely any effort at all, and 10 is maximum effort.

Your six-week
postnatal plan

	Week 1	Week 2	Week 3	Week 4	Week 5	Week 6
Monday	12-Minute Power Pram Walk	12-Minute Power Pram Walk and Postnatal Circuit Weeks 1&2 (p132)	16-Minute Power Pram Walk	Postnatal Circuit Weeks 3&4 (p136)	24-Minute Power Pram Walk	Postnatal Circuit Weeks 5&6 (p140)
Tuesday	Postnatal Circuit Weeks 1&2 (p132)	Rest Day ♥ Treat yourself to an exfoliating body brush (see p54)	Postnatal Circuit Weeks 3&4 (p136)	16-Minute Power Pram Walk	Postnatal Circuit Weeks 5&6 (p140)	24-Minute Power Pram Walk
Wednesday	Postnatal Circuit Weeks 1&2 (p132)	12-Minute Power Pram Walk	16-Minute Power Pram Walk	Postnatal Circuit Weeks 3&4 (p136)	24-Minute Power Pram Walk	Postnatal Circuit Weeks 5&6 (p140)
Thursday	12-Minute Power Pram Walk	Postnatal Circuit Weeks 1&2 (p132)	Rest Day ♥ Pamper yourself with a hair mask (see p108)	16-Minute Power Pram Walk	Postnatal Circuit Weeks 5&6 (p140)	24-Minute Power Pram Walk
Friday	Postnatal Circuit Weeks 1&2 (p132)	Postnatal Circuit Weeks 1&2 (p132)	16-Minute Power Pram Walk	Postnatal Circuit Weeks 3&4 (p136)	24-Minute Power Pram Walk	Postnatal Circuit Weeks 5&6 (p140)
Saturday	12-Minute Power Pram Walk and Postnatal Circuit Weeks 1&2 (p132)	12-Minute Power Pram Walk	Postnatal Circuit Weeks 3&4 (p136)	16-Minute Power Pram Walk and Postnatal Circuit Weeks 3&4 (p136)	Rest Day ♥ Pamper yourself with a face mask (see p72)	24-Minute Power Pram Walk and Postnatal Circuit Weeks 5&6 (p140)
Sunday	Rest Day ♥ Why not treat yourself to a relaxing feel good treat? (see p126)	Postnatal Circuit Weeks 1&2 (p132)	16-Minute Power Pram Walk and Postnatal Circuit Weeks 3&4 (p136)	Rest Day ♥ Pamper yourself with a soothing body wrap (see p90)	24-Minute Power Pram Walk and Postnatal Circuit Weeks 5&6 (p140)	Rest Day ♥ Now you will feel and look fabulous so why not give your new body a special glow? (see p36)

WEEKS 1&2
start gently...

This easy circuit will take less than five minutes to complete, so it's perfect for when your baby is having a short nap. The first exercise will gently increase your core temperature, which means you don't have to worry about doing a warm-up. All three moves will work your pelvic floor, abdominals, bottom and thighs, without overstressing any of them.

Start here ↘

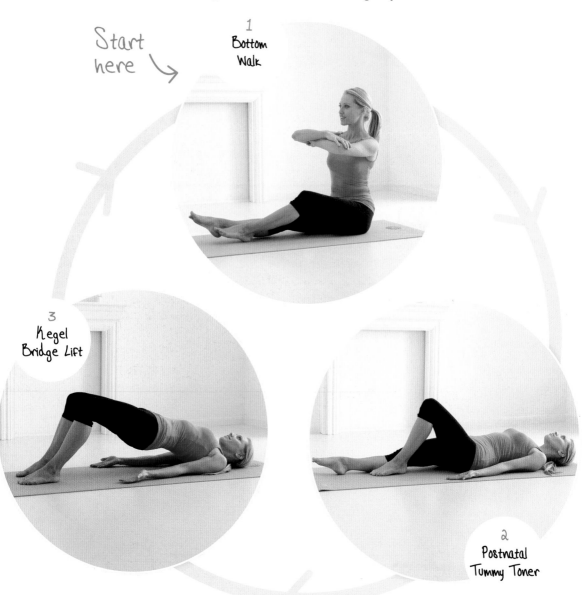

1
Bottom Walk

3
Kegel Bridge Lift

2
Postnatal Tummy Toner

Exercise one

Bottom Walk

What it does
This improves posture, flexibility and helps warm up your body for the other exercises. It will also sculpt your bottom and start work on re-strengthening your abdominal muscles.

How to do it
Sit upright with good posture at the end of your mat, both legs fully extended, and cross your arms at shoulder level. Pull in your abdominals and keep your chin up. Lift one side of your bottom off the floor and slide forward slightly before doing the same on the other side, so you shuffle down the mat. Aim to do 10 lengths of the mat.

Tip
Keeping your tummy pulled in will help to strengthen your deep abdominal muscles, repairing any muscular separation that has occurred during your pregnancy

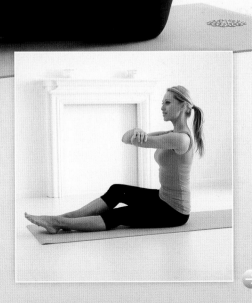

Exercise two

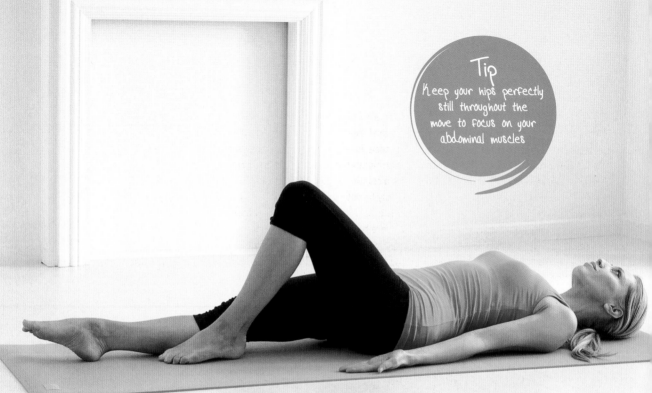

Tip
Keep your hips perfectly still throughout the move to focus on your abdominal muscles

Postnatal Tummy Toner

What it does
This works your transversus abdominis, the deep muscles in your abdomen. It's vital to tackle these muscles in order to repair the linea alba – the tissue down the middle of your abdominals – which gets stretched over the nine months of your pregnancy.

How to do it
Lie face-up on your mat with both your legs extended out straight. Keep your head and shoulders on the floor and put your arms by your sides. Engage your abdominal muscles and slowly bend one knee. Keeping your back flat, slide your heel towards your bottom and back to the start. Make sure you only slide your heel within a range that will keep your back flat on the ground. Do eight on one leg, then repeat on the other side.

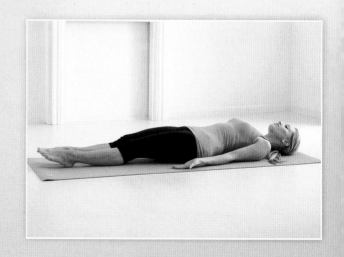

Exercise three

Kegel Bridge Lift

What it does

This simple move targets your abdomen, pelvis, lower back, hips and gluteals (bottom). The addition of the kegel squeeze works your pelvic floor.

How to do it

Lie face-up on your mat with your knees bent and your feet flat on the floor. Keep your head and shoulders on the floor and put your arms by your sides, palms facing up. Slowly raise your hips until your body is straight from knees to shoulders. Now squeeze your buttocks and pull in your abdominals to protect your back, hold for a couple of seconds then lower slowly back to the floor. Engage your pelvic floor muscles by imagining that you are having a pee and you have to hold it (this is your pelvic floor muscles working). Hold for 10 seconds, release and repeat the lift followed by the pelvic floor squeeze. Perform 10 times.

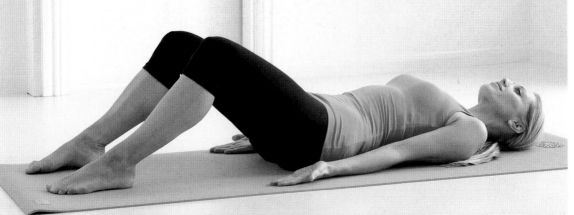

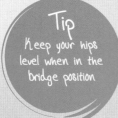

Tip
Keep your hips level when in the bridge position

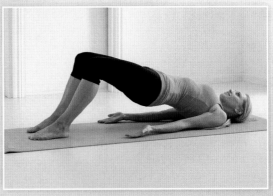

WEEKS 3&4
building up...

Over the next two weeks, you'll continue with the exercises you did in Weeks 1 and 2, only now you'll add three new exercises that will tone your arms, chest, bottom and hips, as well as your deep core muscles. You'll still be able to complete each workout in less than 10 minutes.

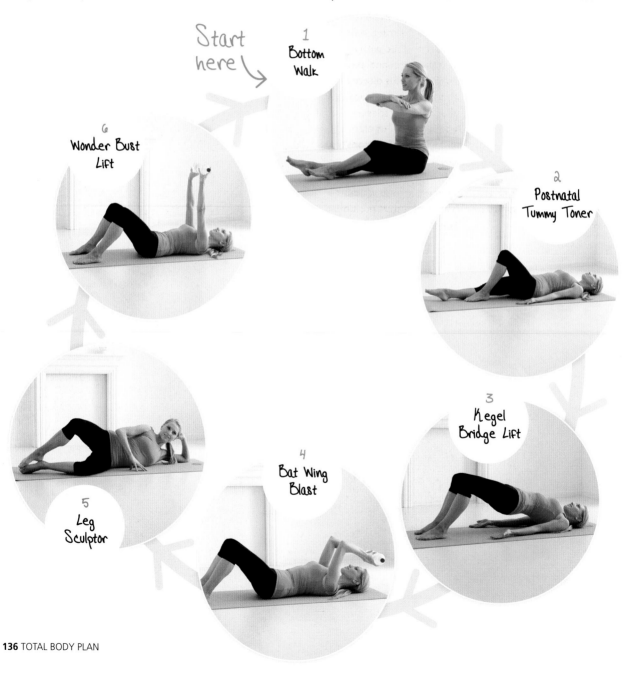

Start here →

1 Bottom Walk

6 Wonder Bust Lift

2 Postnatal Tummy Toner

3 Kegel Bridge Lift

4 Bat Wing Blast

5 Leg Sculptor

Exercise four

Bat Wing Blast

What it does

Tone up the backs of your arms – technically referred to as triceps, but better known as bat wings or bingo wings. Picking up your baby uses the front of your arms, so this will balance things out.

How to do it

For this exercise, you'll need a light dumbbell (2kg) or you can simply use a full bottle of water.

Lie face-up on the mat with both your knees bent and your feet flat on the floor. Hold the bottle with an overhand grip and extend both your arms directly above your face. Brace your abdominal muscles and slowly bend your elbows (take up to four seconds), keeping your upper arms still. Hold for a couple of seconds, then slowly push back to the start position. Repeat 10 times.

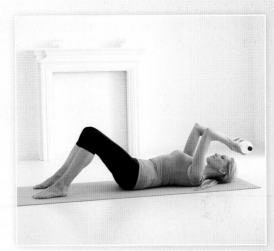

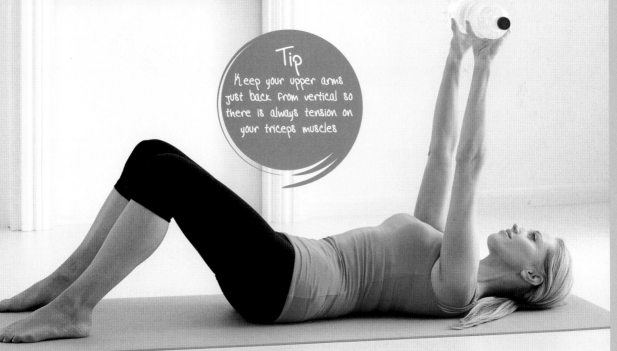

Tip
Keep your upper arms just back from vertical so there is always tension on your triceps muscles

137

Exercise five

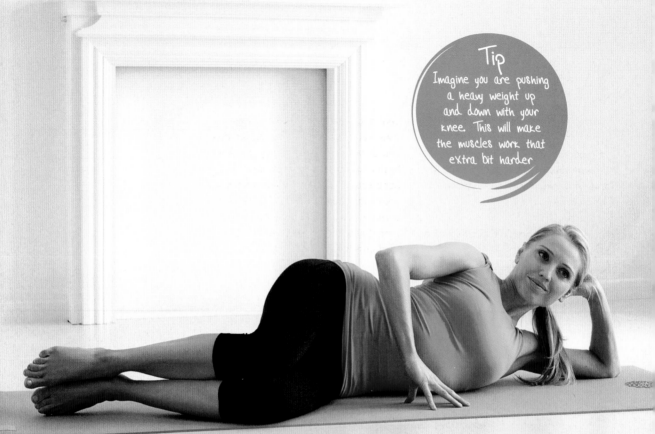

Tip
Imagine you are pushing a heavy weight up and down with your knee. This will make the muscles work that extra bit harder

Leg Sculptor

What it does
This tones and sculpts your thighs and bottom, and also works your deep core muscles by engaging them to stabilise your upper body.

How to do it
Lie on your side on your mat with your head supported on one hand. Keep your heels together and bend your knees to 45°. Keep your spine in its natural alignment with your tummy muscles pulled in. Now slowly lift the top knee, keeping your feet together and rotating from the hip. Hold for a second and lower slowly to the start. Do 10 on each side.

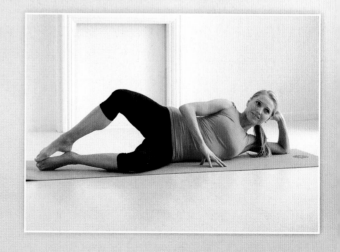

Exercise six

Wonder Bust Lift

What it does

You'll lift your bust by strengthening your pectorals – the muscles that support your chest. You'll shape your arms and shoulders at the same time.

How to do it

Use a dumbbell or a full bottle of water. Lie face-up on your mat with your knees bent and feet flat on the floor. Hold your weight or bottle with hands either end, so your palms are facing up. Extend both arms above your chest. Slowly bend your elbows to the sides and lower the weight (take up to four seconds) towards your chest, hold for a second, then slowly extend arms back to the start position. Repeat 10 times.

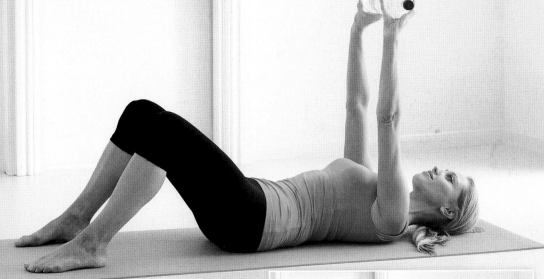

Tip
Add an abs element to this move by pulling your belly button in towards your spine as you lower your arms and again as you push back up

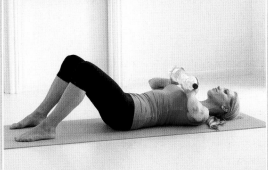

139

WEEKS 5&6
finishing touches...

For this circuit, exercise one works as your warm-up and then you'll target your tummy, bottom, hips, thighs, arms and waist with the other exercises. By the end of the second week, you should be getting back to your best pre-pregnancy shape. After each circuit, spend a few minutes doing some stretching – see p19 for details.

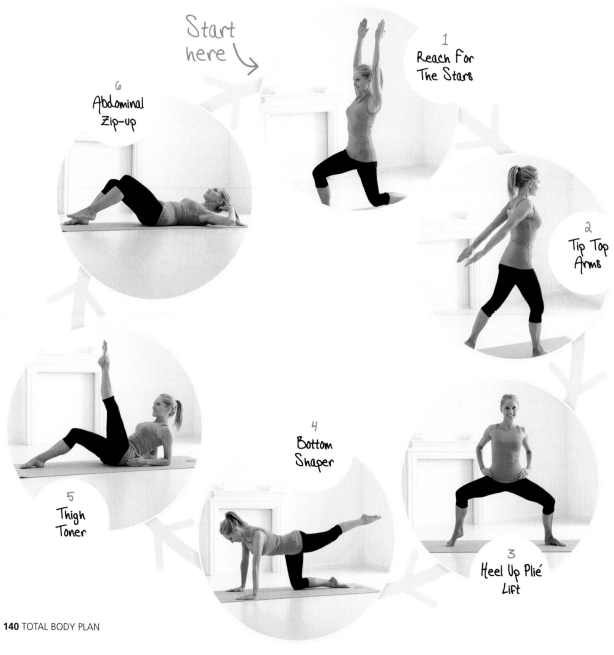

Start here ↘

1 Reach For The Stars

2 Tip Top Arms

3 Heel Up Plié Lift

4 Bottom Shaper

5 Thigh Toner

6 Abdominal Zip-up

Exercise one

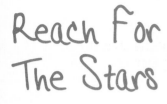

Reach For The Stars

What it does

This dynamic move works your upper body and lower body at the same time. It's great for shaping your thighs, bottom, shoulders and arms, and it will also warm up your core temperature for the other exercises.

How to do it

Stand in a split stance – one foot forward and one foot back – with both feet pointing forwards. Keep your abdominals tight and your body upright throughout the exercise. Bend your knees, keeping your front knee over your front foot, and lower your back knee towards the floor. Extend both your arms above your head as you lower. Return slowly to the start. Do 10 on each side.

Tip
Don't lock out your knees when your legs are straight

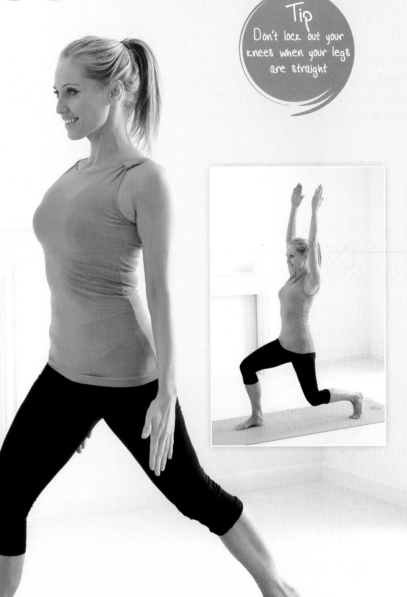

141

Exercise two

Tip Top Arms

What it does

This works on toning your upper arms, and will give you beautiful definition through your arms and shoulders.

How to do it

Stand with your feet in a split stance, keeping your knees soft. Engage your abdominal muscles to support good upper body posture, turn your palms out so they are facing behind you and slowly lift both arms up and away from your body. Hold at the highest point for a couple of seconds (this is a fairly small move – your arms should be about 45° to your body) and slowly lower back to the start. Repeat 16 times.

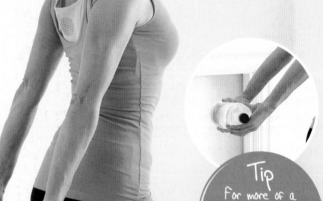

Tip
For more of a challenge, hold a full water bottle in your hands

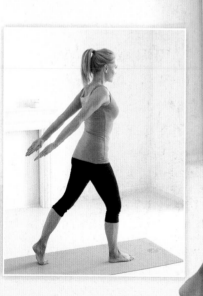

Exercise three

Heel Up Plié Lift

What it does

This is a great way of sculpting and toning your hips, legs and bottom. You'll also target those hard-to-reach inner thighs.

How to do it

Stand with your feet wide apart and have your toes pointing out to a 45° angle. Place your hands on your hips and keep your body upright, with your tummy muscles pulled in. Lift one heel off the floor. Slowly bend your knees, keeping your knees in line with your toes. Hold for a couple of seconds and slowly push back up to the start. Do 10 on each side.

> **Tip**
> If you feel confident of your balance and want a new challenge, do this with both heels lifted at the same time

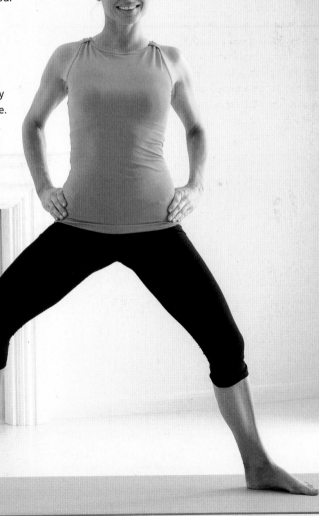

143

Exercise four

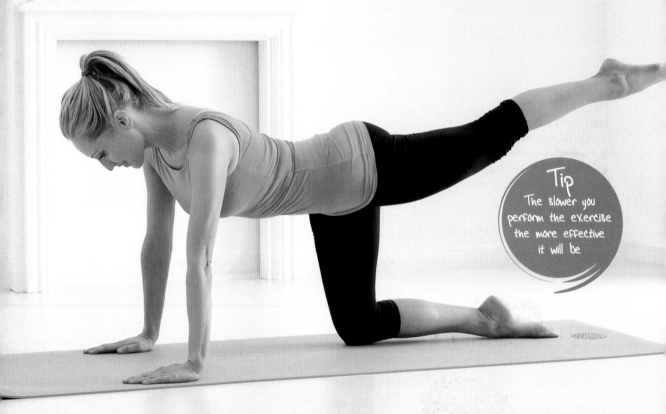

Tip
The slower you perform the exercise the more effective it will be

Bottom Shaper

What it does
This will give your postnatal tummy muscles a deep abdominal workout, and help to lift your gluteus maximus (your bum).

How to do it
Use a mat or towel to protect your knees. Kneel on all-fours, keeping your hands beneath your shoulders and your knees directly under your hips. Pull your belly button into your spine and extend one leg out behind you in line with your hip. Hold for a second and slowly pull your knee in towards your chest, hold for a second then slowly extend back out. Repeat 10 times on this leg, then change to the other leg and repeat 10 times.

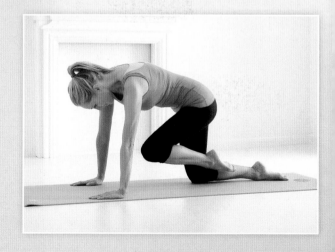

Exercise five

Thigh Toner

What it does
This exercise manages to be relaxing and challenging at the same time. It will tone your thighs while stretching out your hamstrings and glutes.

How to do it
Lie on your mat and lean back on your forearms with both hands pointing forwards. Bend one knee and extend the other leg out in front of you. Keep your chin parallel to the floor and pull your belly button in towards your spine. Slowly lift your extended leg off the floor, bringing it as high as you comfortably can without letting it bend at the knee. Hold for a second then slowly lower back down. Do 10 repetitions on each side.

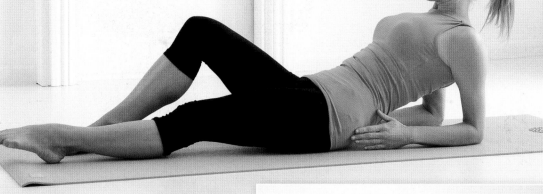

Tip
For an extra challenge sit up higher. This instantly makes the thigh movement harder.

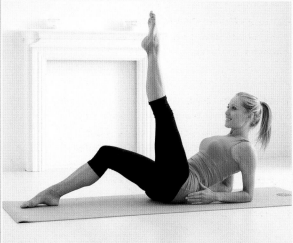

Exercise six

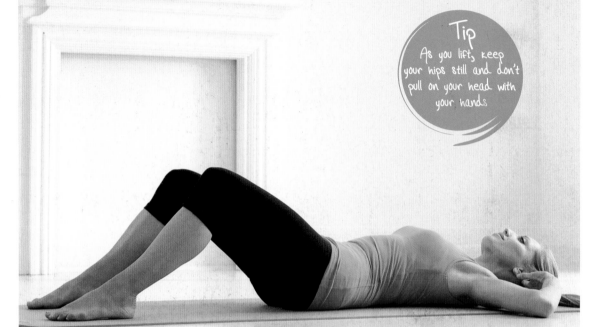

Cayenne Goddess Top, £65.95, wellicious.com; Vintage Rose Divine yoga mat with Swarovski Elements, £149, wellicious.com. Shot at the Wellicious yoga studio in London.

Tip
As you lift, keep your hips still and don't pull on your head with your hands

Abdominal Zip-up

What it does

This is a great postnatal exercise because it engages all your abdominal muscles in one move without any jerky or uncomfortable actions that might cause injury.

How to do it

Lie face-up on your mat with both knees bent and your feet flat on the floor. Place your hands by your ears and keep your elbows in line with your shoulders. Look up towards the ceiling. Take a deep breath in and slowly breathe out as you lift your head and shoulders off the floor – making sure you keep your tummy muscles pulled in tight – and at the same time, lift one foot just slightly off the floor. Hold for a second, then slowly lower to the start. Repeat 10 times, alternating feet with each rep.

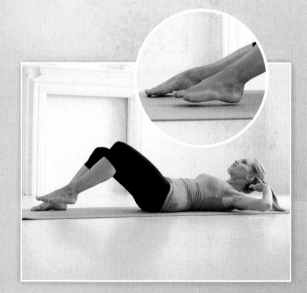